Gene Editing - Technologies and Applications

Edited by Yuan-Chuan Chen and Shiu-Jau Chen

Published in London, United Kingdom

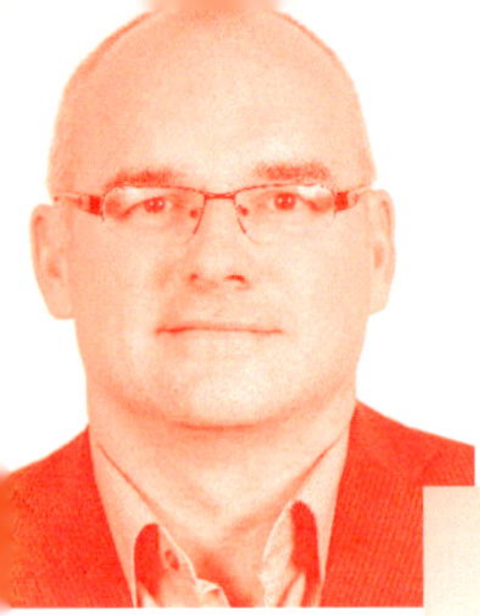
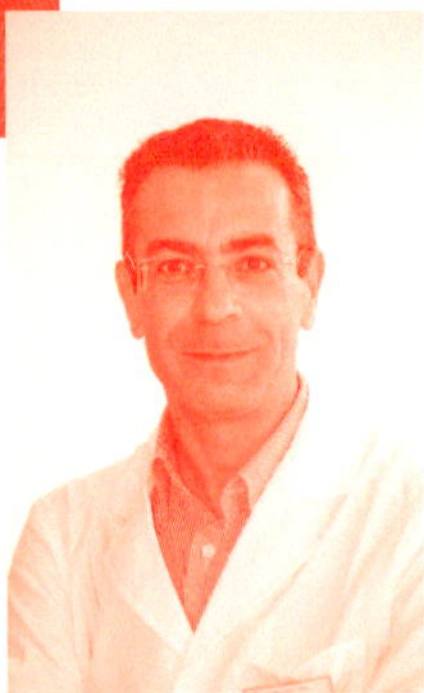
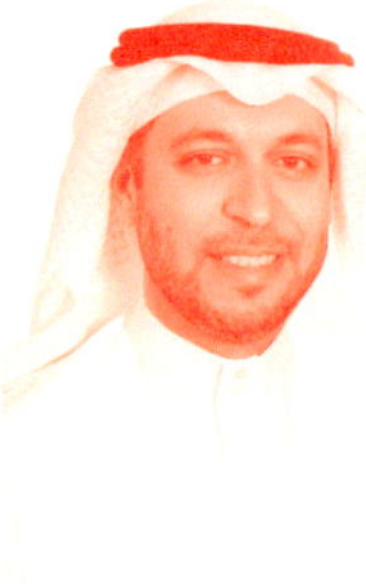
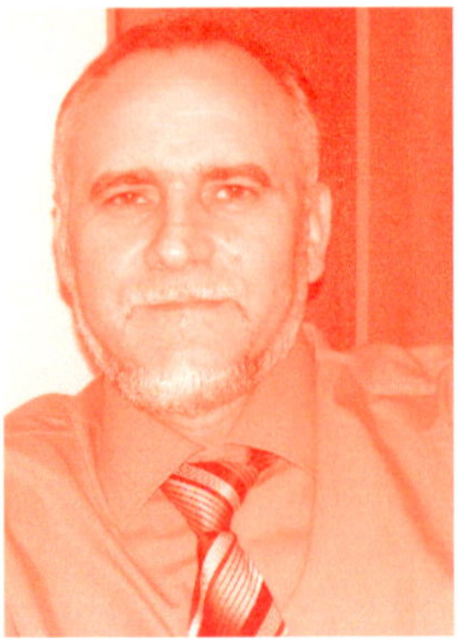
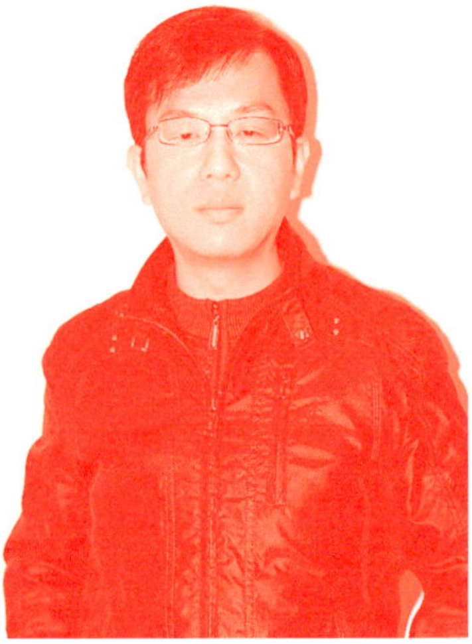
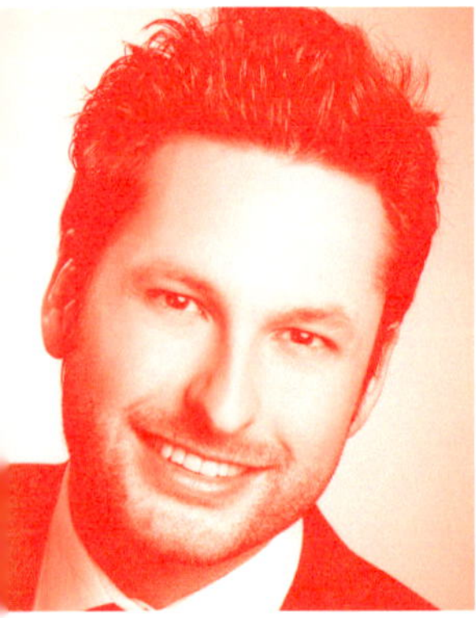
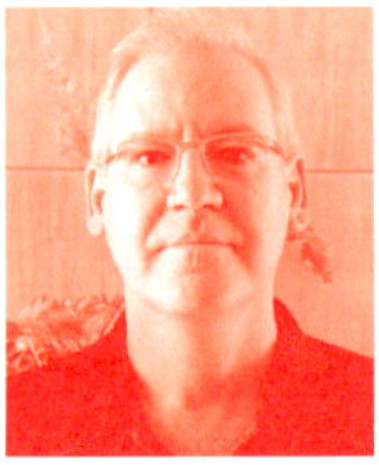

IntechOpen

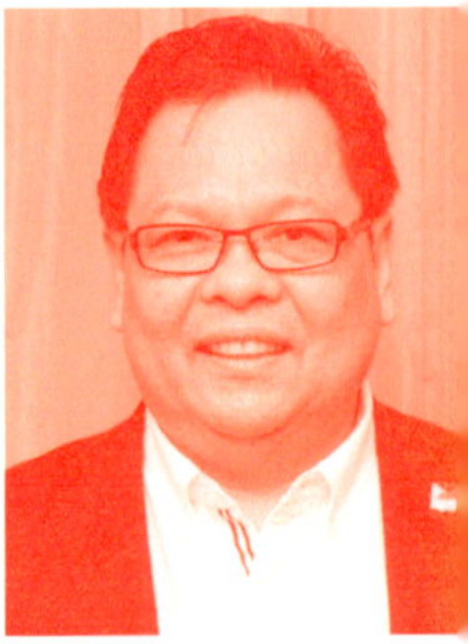
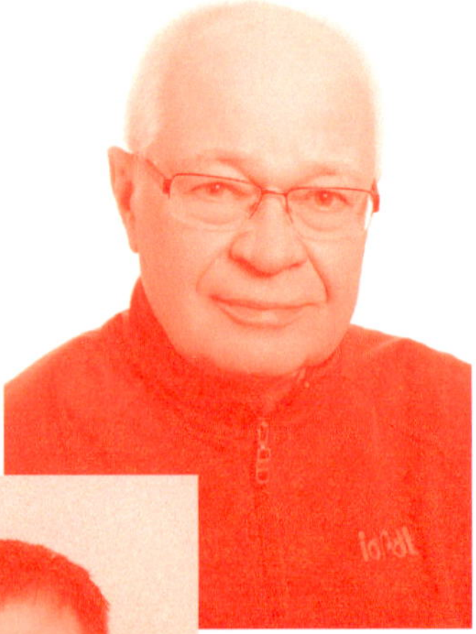
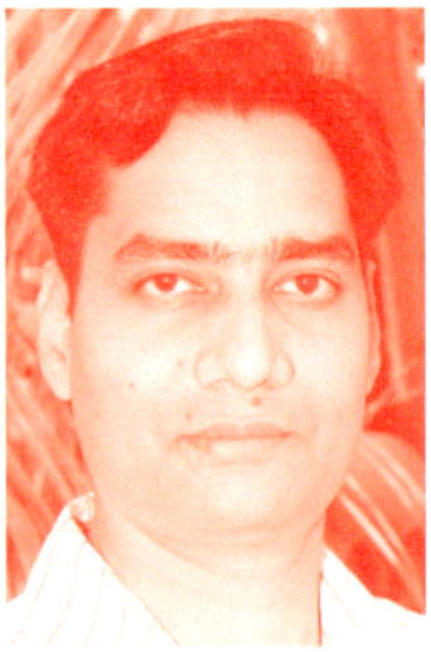
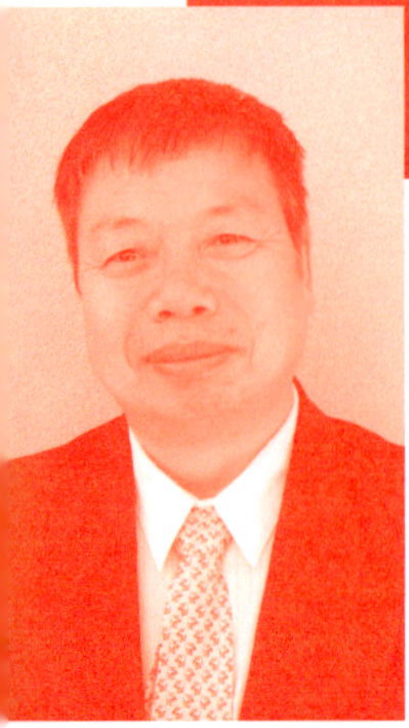
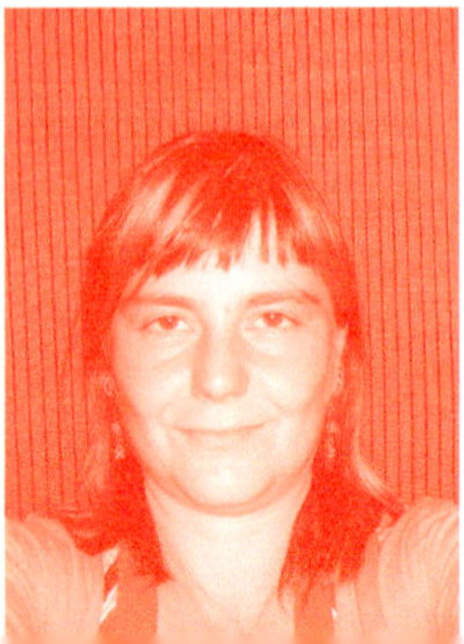
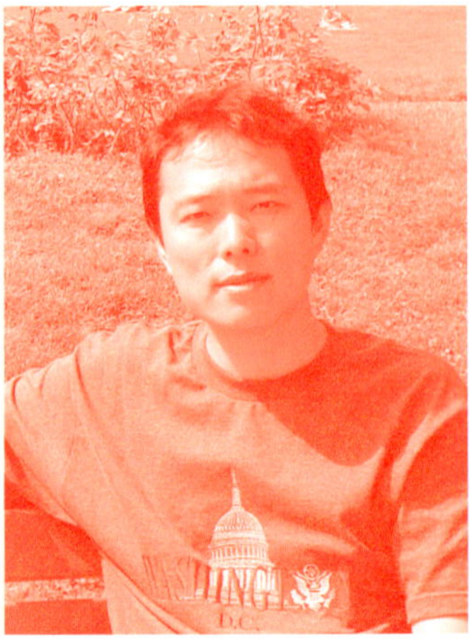

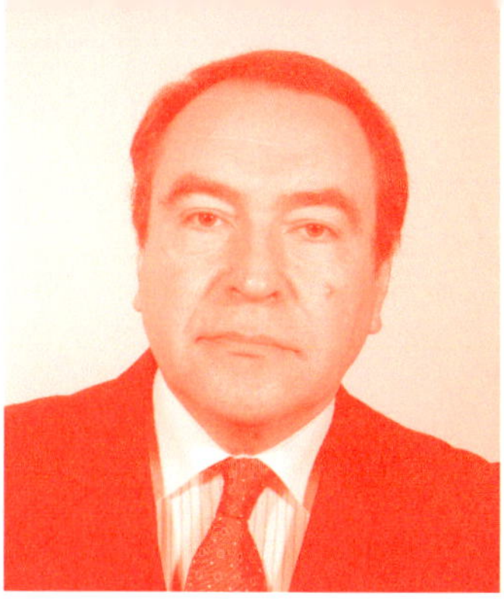
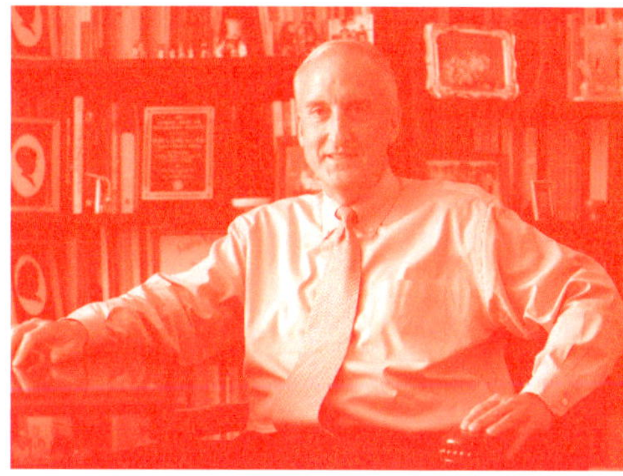
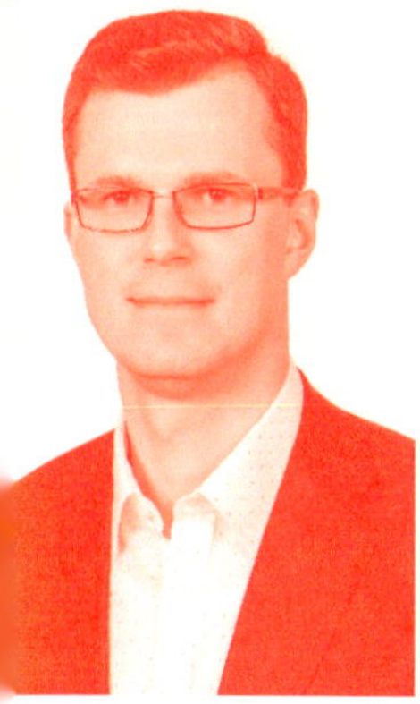
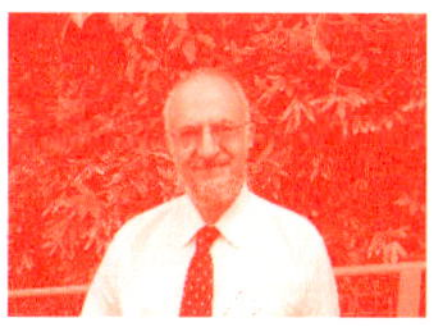
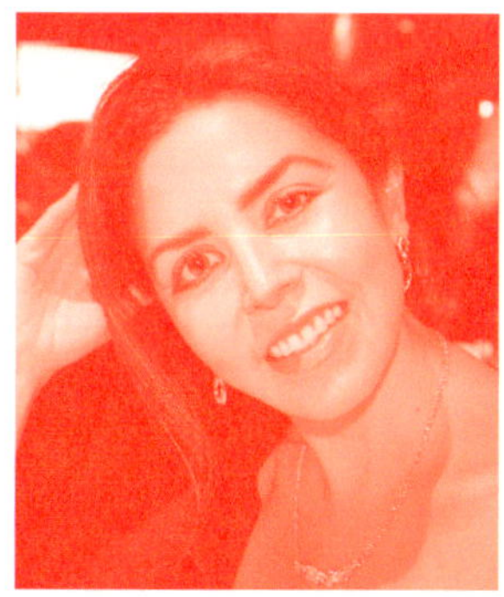

Supporting open minds since 2005

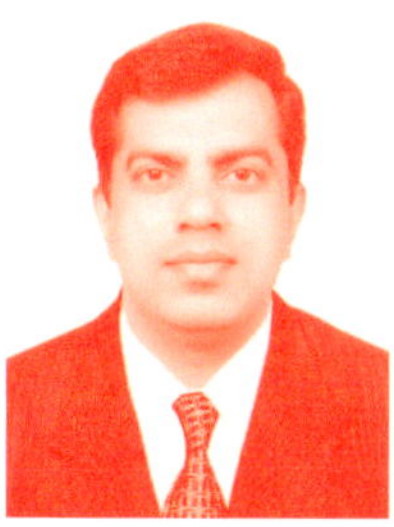
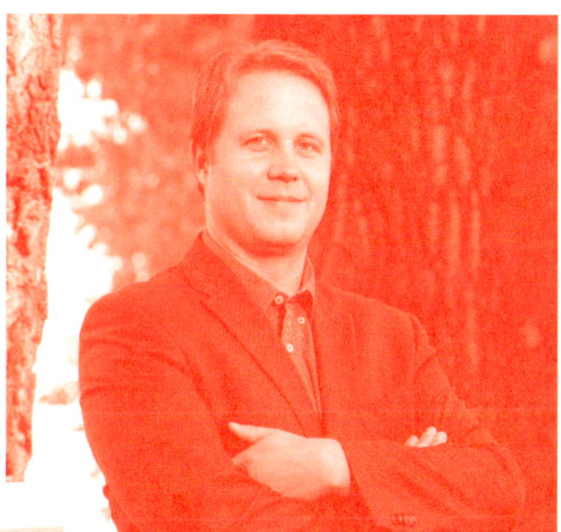
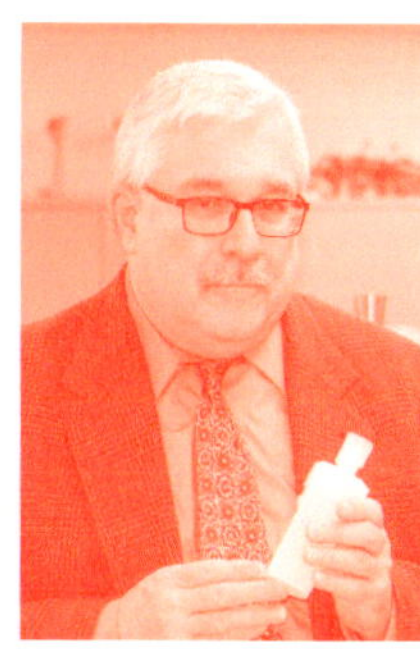
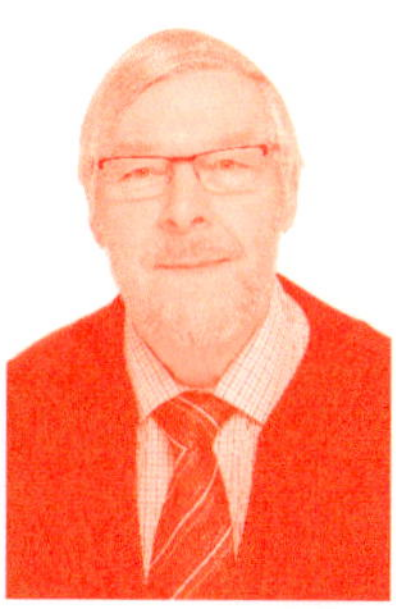
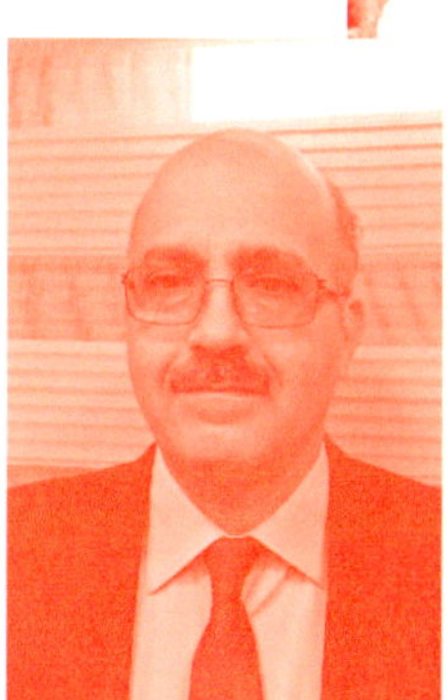
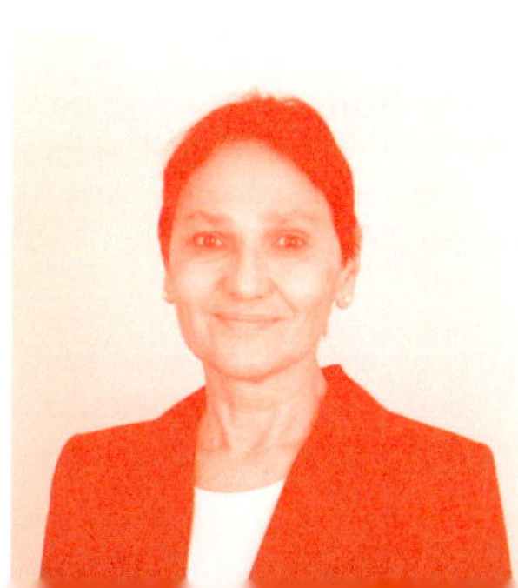
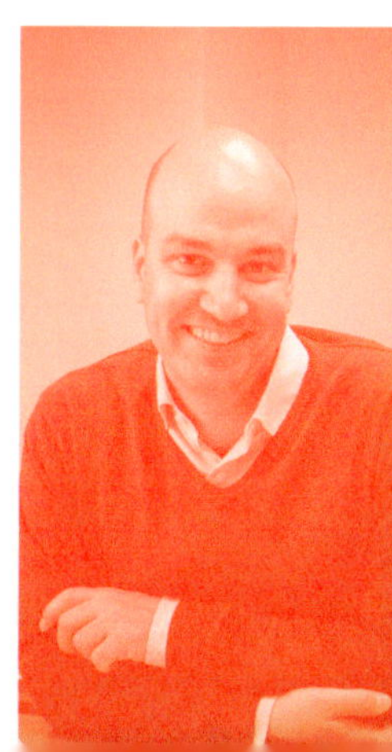

Gene Editing - Technologies and Applications
http://dx.doi.org/10.5772/intechopen.82127
Edited by Yuan-Chuan Chen and Shiu-Jau Chen

Contributors
Shahid Nazir, Muhammad Zaffar Iqbal, Sajid-Ur-Rahman, Masahiro Sato, Shingo Nakamura, Huafeng Lin, Qiudi Deng, Lei Shi, Yuan-Chuan Chen

First published in London, United Kingdom, 2019 by IntechOpen
IntechOpen is the global imprint of INTECHOPEN LIMITED, registered in England and Wales, registration number: 11086078, The Shard, 25th floor, 32 London Bridge Street
London, SE19SG - United Kingdom
Printed in Croatia

British Library Cataloguing-in-Publication Data
A catalogue record for this book is available from the British Library

Additional hard and PDF copies can be obtained from orders@intechopen.com

Gene Editing - Technologies and Applications
Edited by Yuan-Chuan Chen and Shiu-Jau Chen
p. cm.
Print ISBN 978-1-78984-508-2
Online ISBN 978-1-78984-509-9
eBook (PDF) ISBN 978-1-83880-689-7

For EU product safety concerns:
IN TECH d.o.o., Prolaz Marije Krucifikse Kozulić 3, 51000 Rijeka, Croatia, info@intechopen.com or visit our website at intechopen.com.

Meet the editors

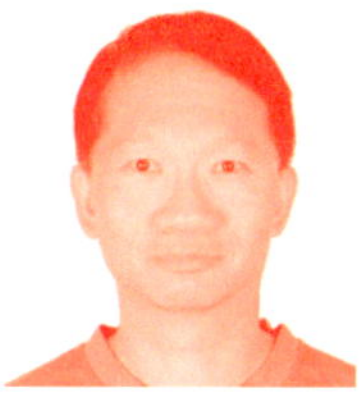

Yuan-Chuan Chen completed his PhD in Biochemistry at the University of California, Berkeley, USA, in 2015. His research interests include pharmacy/pharmacology, biochemistry, microbiology/virology, cell/molecule biology, biotechnology/nanotechnology, cell/gene therapy, and policy/regulation. His studies focus on the discovery, application, perspectives, and challenges of biopharmaceuticals. Additionally, he is interested in basic research, multiple applications, and human therapeutics using CRISPR/Cas9.

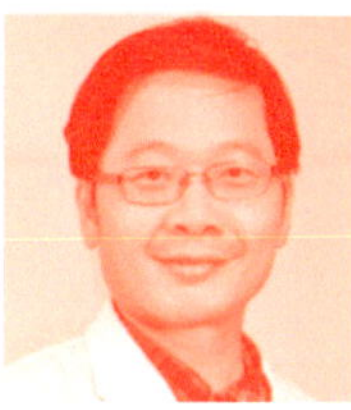

Shiu-Jau Chen obtained his medical doctor (MD) degree and completed his PhD in Anatomy and Cell Biology at the National Taiwan University in 1994 and 2013, respectively. His specialty is neurosurgery and brain disease treatment. His studies focus on the prevention and treatment of drug addiction and neurodegenerative diseases. He is also interested in the treatment of Parkinson's disease and Alzheimer's disease using CRISPR/Cas9.

Contents

Preface

For conventional genetic cloning, target genes are cleaved at restriction sites using restriction endonucleases. Researchers cannot modify genomic sites and it usually takes a lot of work, time, and patience to make and screen for desired clones. Current gene-editing technologies, including ZFNs, TALENs, and CRISPRs/Cas9, can be utilized to engineer the genes of interest in living organisms with unprecedented efficiency and precision, without the limitation of restriction site availability. Specific and efficient genomic engineering has been performed in human cells, microbes, plants, animals, etc. at will. Additionally, it has been applied in manufacturing products, including testing tools, agricultural products, foods, industrial products, medicinal products, etc. Among them, novel therapeutic strategies based on gene-editing technologies are expected to bring hope for patient recovery from serious diseases for which there are still no effective drugs or medical devices available.

Many biotechnology companies have successfully produced nonhuman therapeutic products and medicinal products using gene-editing technologies. More and more products are being developed and approved for sale. Consequently, many enterprises are encouraged to become involved in manufacturing products based on these technologies because of their perspectives for multiple applications. For example, CRISPR has become an industry that is developing prosperously. These enterprises also promote industry innovation through the transfer of technologies and collaboration between academia and industry.

Gene-editing technologies are still being discovered and are expected to become more mature, specific, efficient, and secure for applications in the near future. The potential benefits of these revolutionary technologies are endless. However, like any powerful tool, there are also associated challenges, including safety and ethical/moral concerns, that need to be considered. Research and ethical guidelines from national and international organizations will be critical for funding agencies and institutional review boards to regulate these technologies, especially in the gene editing of human germ line cells and embryos. The aim is to maximize the benefits and minimize the possible risks of gene-editing technologies.

We wish all current and future research work, including the discovery, applications, perspectives, and challenges of gene-editing technologies, to have a worthwhile impact on the betterment of human health. It is hoped that all perspectives will become realities and any challenges will be overcome provided that academia, industry, governments, and international societies constantly endeavor and cooperate with each other. Finally, we are grateful for all authors' participation and IntechOpen's enthusiasm in helping us to complete and publish this book.

Yuan-Chuan Chen, PhD
Program in Comparative Biochemistry,
University of California,
Berkeley, CA, USA

Shiu-Jau Chen, MD, PhD
Department of Neurosurgery,
Mackay Memorial Hospital,
Taipei, Taiwan

Section 1

Background

Chapter 1

Introductory Chapter: Gene Editing Technologies and Applications

Yuan-Chuan Chen

1. Introduction

Gene editing is a type of genetic engineering in which DNA is inserted, deleted, modified, or replaced in the genome of a living organism. Unlike traditional methods that randomly insert genetic material into a host genome, current gene editing technologies target and change the specific genome locations. Zinc finger nucleases (ZFNs), transcription activator-like effectors nucleases (TALENs), and clustered regularly interspaced short palindromic repeats (CRISPRs)/Cas9 nuclease system are the three common gene editing technologies. These technologies have been widely used in genome engineering to enable a broad range of mutation by inducing DNA breaks that stimulate error-prone repairs such as homologous recombination (HR) or nonhomologous end joining (NHEJ). They successfully make it possible to achieve site-specific editing, modification, and manipulation at specific genomic sites (**Table 1**) [1].

1.1 ZFNs

ZFNs are artificial restriction enzymes generated by fusing a zinc finger-specific DNA-binding domain to a nonspecific DNA cleavage domain. The specific binding domains of individual ZFNs typically contain between three and six individual zinc finger repeats and can each recognize between 12 and 18 base pairs. If the zinc finger domains are specific for their intended target site, then even a pair of three-finger ZFNs that recognize a total of 18 base pairs can target a single locus in a mammalian genome. The nonspecific cleavage domain from the restriction endonuclease *Fok I* is typically used as the cleavage domain in ZFNs. This cleavage domain must form a dimer in order to cleave DNA, and thus a pair of ZFNs are required to target nonpalindromic DNA sites [2] (**Figure 1**).

1.2 TALENs

Transcription activator-like effectors (TALEs) are proteins secreted by bacteria *Xanthomonas* via type III secretion system when they infect various plant species. TALEs are important virulence factors that act as transcriptional activators in the plant cell nucleus [3]. Each TALE contains a central repetitive region consisting of varying numbers of repeat units (about 17.5 repeats) of 34 amino acids [3, 4]. The DNA-binding domain contains a highly conserved 34 amino acid sequence with the exception of the 12th and 13th amino acids [3]. Only the 12th and 13th amino acids in TALEs are changeable and variable, the other amino acids are constant and

Technology	ZFN	TALEN	CRISPR/Cas9
Source	Extensively exists in the nature	Plant pathogenic bacteria *Xanthomonas*	An adaptive immune system in bacteria
Targeting specificity determinant	Zinc finger protein	TALE	SgRNA
Nuclease	*Fok* I	*Fok* I	Cas9
Restriction for a target sequence	Rich in cytosine	No special restriction	PAM
Target site	Two (left and right)	Two (left and right)	Only one
Length of target gene	12–18 bp	12–18 bp	18–23 bp
Mode of action	Two proteins act on two target sites	Two proteins act on two target sites	RNA and Cas9 act on one target site
Cleavage site	DSB with a sticky end	DSB with a sticky end	DSB with a blunt end
Efficiency	Medium	Medium	High
Ease of engineering	Low	Medium	High
Ease of characterization	Low	Medium	High
Cost	High	Medium	Low
Cytotoxicity	High	Low	Low
Off target	Yes	Yes	Yes

Abbreviations: CRISPR, clustered regularly interspaced short palindromic repeat; DSB, double-strand break; Fok, Flavobacterium okeanokoites; PAM, protospacer adjacent motif; TALE, transcription activator-like effector; sgRNA, single guide RNA; and ZFN, zinc finger nuclease.

Table 1.
Comparison of different gene editing technologies.

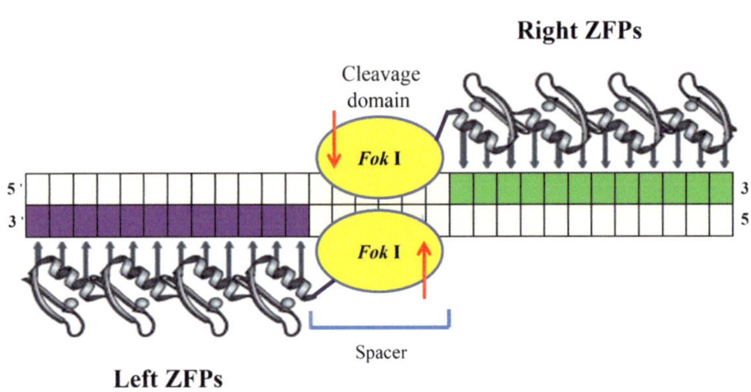

Figure 1.
ZFNs are chimeric nucleases consisting of specific DNA-binding modules linked to a nonspecific cleavage domain. Right and left ZFNs containing Fok I endonucleases link to an array of 3–6 zinc fingers that have been designed to specifically recognize target sequences (12 green and 12 purple boxes), respectively. The ZFN targets are separated by typically 5 or 6 bp. Two Fok I work as a homodimer to cleave the sense strand 1 bp and antisense strand 5 bp downstream of the binding site.

stable. These two locations—repeat variable di-residues (RVD) are highly variable and show a strong correlation with a specific nucleotide recognition by different frequency, for example, NI recognize A (55%), NG recognize T (50%), NN recognize G (7%), and HD recognize C(69%) [3]. Two amino acids have known to recognize one nucleotide after the breaking of code of DNA-binding specificity of

TALEs [3, 4]. The restriction endonuclease *Fok* I consists of an N-terminal specific DNA-binding domain and a C-terminal nonspecific DNA cleavage domain. The nonspecific DNA cleavage domain of *Fok* I cleaves the double-strand DNA (DSB) at a fixed distance of 9 and 13 nucleotides downstream of the recognition site [5]. TALENs are artificial restriction enzymes generated by fusing the specific TALE DNA-binding domain to a nonspecific *Fok* I DNA cleavage domain [6–8] (**Figure 2**).

1.3 CRISPRs/Cas9

The CRISPRs/Cas9 system, originally found in the bacteria, functions as an adaptive immune system against foreign virus or plasmid DNA. CRISPRs are DNA loci containing short repetitions of base sequences. Each repetition is followed by short segments of spacer DNA from previous exposures to the foreign DNA. CRISPR-associated protein (Cas9) is a DNA endonuclease whose structure is bilobed, composed of target recognition domain and nuclease lobes. The nuclease

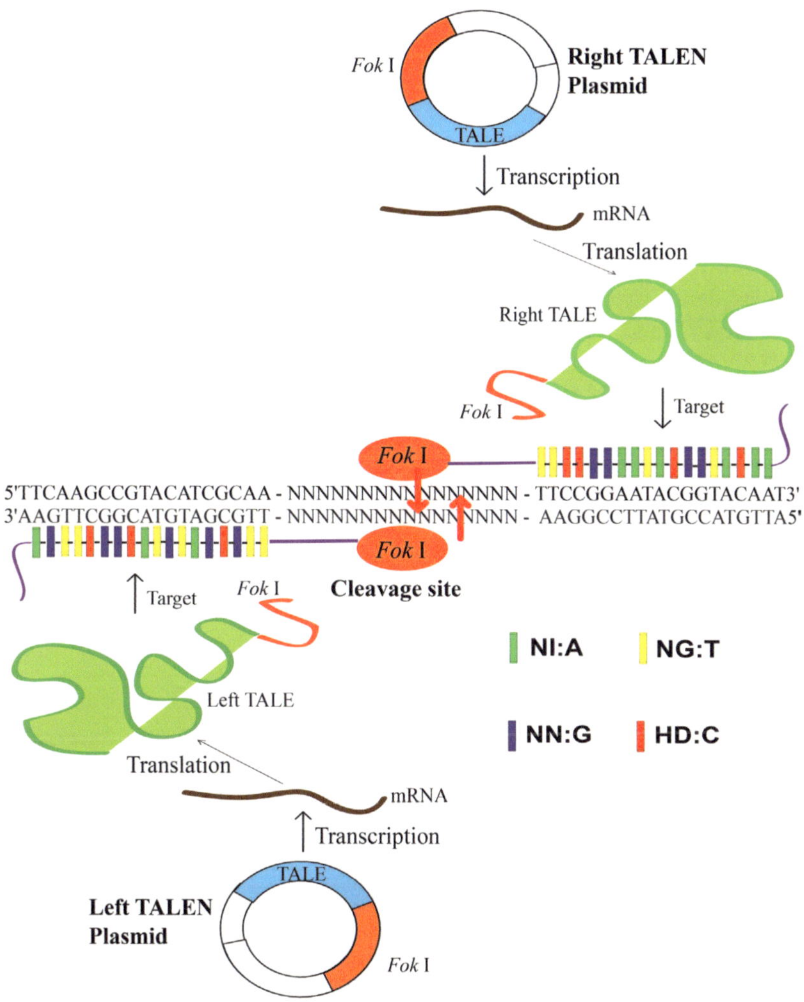

Figure 2.
The specific repeat variable Di-residues (RVDs) used to recognize each base are defined in the key (NI:A, NG:T, NN:G, and HD:C). Left and right TALEs recognize their target sequences and allow their associated Fok I endonucleases to work as a homodimer to cleave the sense strand 9 bp and antisense strand 13 bp downstream of the binding site. Binding of TALEs to the target sites allows Fok I to dimerize and create a double-strand break (DSB) with sticky ends within the spacer.

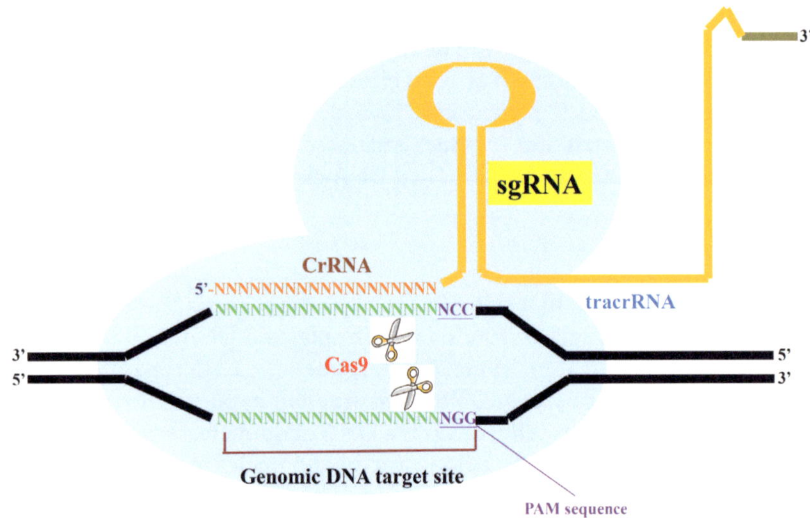

Figure 3.
A crRNA/tracrRNA hybrid acts as a single guide RNA (sgRNA) to recognize their target sequences and allow Cas9 endonucleases to cleave the sense strand 3 bp and antisense strand 3 bp upstream of the protospacer adjacent motif (PAM) sequence. Binding of sgRNAs to the target sites makes Cas9 create a double-strand break (DSB) with blunt ends on target sequences.

lobe contains nucleases RuvC, HNH, and a carboxyl-terminal domain for the protospacer adjacent motif (PAM) recognition [9]. The Type II CRISPRs system is currently limited to target sequences that are N12-20NGG, where NGG represents the PAM sequence [10]. Any potential target sequence must have a specific PAM sequence on its 3′ end. The CRISPR locus consists of Cas9 endonucleases, CRISPRs RNAs (crRNAs), trans-activating crRNAs (tracrRNAs), and precursor crRNAs (pre-crRNAs). tracrRNA is partially complementary to and pairs with a pre-crRNA to form an RNA duplex cleaved by RNase III. The crRNA/tracrRNA hybrid acts as a single guide RNA (sgRNA) for the Cas9, which cleaves the invading DNA. The DNA target sites can appear in multiple locations, all of which will be targeted by the Cas9 for cleavage. By delivering the Cas9 protein and appropriate sgRNAs into a cell, the organism's genome can be cut at most locations with the only limitation of PAM availability (**Figure 3**).

2. Application

2.1 Tools for basic research

2.1.1 Genetic cloning of living organisms

For conventional genetic cloning of animals, plants, and microbes, the target genes in the specific genome are cut using restriction enzymes. It usually takes lots of work and long time to clone and screen for the desired ones. Current gene editing technologies can be used to achieve the desired clones both quickly and accurately, without the limitation of restriction site availability [11].

2.1.2 Establishment of animal models

Genetic cloning, gene knock-in, and gene knockout are the most common methods to make induced or experimental animal models. The efficient approaches include ZFNs, TALENs, and CRISPRs/Cas9. By these new gene editing technologies, specific animal models of many diseases for which there are no animal models available previously have been established with unprecedented efficiency and precision [12–14].

2.1.3 Development of testing tools and reagents

CRISPRs/Cas9 can be optimized by bacterial genotypes to be more adaptive to the variation of food pathogens, compared with traditional methods. The CRISPR locus of different bacterial species show high variance to be an ideal basis for genotyping [15]. The CRISPR/Cas12a(Cpf1) DETECTR (DNA endonuclease targeted CRISPR trans reporter) system can be used to diagnose gene mutations, cancers, and microbial infections and test microbial antibiotic resistance by analyzing specimens [16].

2.1.4 Discovery of drugs

The screening and identification of target sites are critical to drug discovery; thus, excellent and suitable platforms are needed. Gene editing technologies can work for the editing of functional genes and the screening of target sites. For example, CRISPRs/Cas9 was used to target the exons encoding functional protein domains. A screen of 192 chromatin regulatory domains in murine acute myeloid leukemia (AML) cells identified 6 known drug targets and 19 additional dependencies [17].

2.2 Nonhuman therapeutics

2.2.1 Agricultural products

The gene editing technology can be used to produce agricultural products in accordance with the need of humans. For example, crops were produced with high yield and resistant to diseases, insects, herbicides, and harsh environment [18, 19]; domesticated animals (pig, buffalo) were produced with double muscle phenotype [20]; and aquatic products (catfish) were produced with high level myostatin (MSTN) gene expression [21].

2.2.2 Food

We can make food more productive or have longer shelf-life by gene editing technologies. For example, CRISPRs/Cas9 was used to edit thermophilic bacteria *Streptococcus thermophilus* as a bacteriophage-insensitive mutant to improve the product (e.g., yogurt, cheese) yield by refraining from the infection of phages [22]. The white button mushroom *Agaricus bisporus* was engineered to resist browning using CRISPRs/Cas9. The effect was achieved by targeting to knock out the genes that encodes polyphenol oxidase—an enzyme that causes browning [23].

2.2.3 Industrial products

CRISPRs/Cas9 has been used to establish marine algae (e.g., diatoms) as useful in industrial applications as the carbon neutral synthesis of fuels, pharmaceuticals, health foods, biomolecules, materials related to nanotechnology, and bioremediations of contaminated water [24, 25]. CRISPRs/Cas9 was used to encode the pixel values of black and white images and a short movie into the living bacterial genomes. By CRISPRs/Cas9, the technical limits of this information storage system can be optimized to be minimal. CRISPRs/Cas9 can capture and stably store many real data within the genomes of living cells [26].

2.2.4 Environmental protection

Marine microalgae are in charge of about 40% of primary production on earth and capture more CO_2 than rain forests. Diatoms are the most important unicellular eukaryotic microalgae and have dominant ecological significance. CRISPRs/Cas9 can be used to modify the diatom genome to achieve more effects in reducing the global warming [25].

2.2.5 Restoration of extinct animals

Woolly mammoths are different from current living elephants by adapting to the extreme cold environment. The mammoth TRPV3 gene, which encodes a temperature-sensitive transient receptor potential (thermoTRP) channel involved in thermal sensation and hair growth, could be achieved by modifying genes of Asian elephants [27]. The mammoth may be restored using CRISPRs/Cas9, if the modified embryo can be successfully transferred into the uterus of living elephants.

2.3 Human therapeutics

2.3.1 Medicine screening

The therapeutic strategies of Parkinson's disease (PD) are quite variable including drug and nondrug treatment. Therefore, it is necessary to find a suitable strategy to treat PD safely, efficiently, and quickly. A novel tool was established for monitoring endogenous alpha-synuclein (α-SYN) transcription by NanoLuc luciferase tag insertion at the 3′ end using CRISPRs/Cas9, and thus making it possible to screen for strategies rapidly that can be used for PD therapy efficiently [28].

2.3.2 Preparation for cell therapy or immunotherapy

The gene-editing technology can be applied to engineer induced pluripotent stem (iPS) cells and chimeric antigen receptor T (CART) cells. CRISPRs/Cas9 has been used to engineer iPS cells to evade immune rejection in full immunocompetent allogeneic recipients [29]. Because the CD19 CAR was successfully used in treatment, CRISPRs/Cas9 may further enhance the efficacy and safety of CART cells by engineering therapeutic T cells [30].

2.3.3 Potential application for disease treatment

2.3.3.1 Virus latent infection

Diseases caused by viruses are difficult to treat due to their high mutation rates and latent infections. It is almost impossible to eradicate latent viruses in the human host. However, TALENs and CRISPRs/Cas9 have been found to provide good strategies in targeting viruses and limiting their productive and latent infections *ex vivo* and/or *in vivo*, such as herpes simplex virus 1 (HSV-1), Epstein-Barr virus (EBV), human cytomegalovirus (HCMV), human immunodeficiency virus (HIV), and hepatitis B virus (HBV) [31–36].

2.3.3.2 Genetic disease

Genetic diseases can be cured by gene therapies such as sickle cell anemia, β-thalassemia, muscular dystrophy, α1-antitrypsin deficiency, Leber congenital amaurosis, and cystic fibrosis [37]. The gene editing technologies (e.g., CRISPRs/Cas9) potentially facilitate the progress of gene therapy, because many experiments have been successful *ex vivo* and *in vivo*, and some of them are being under clinical trials.

2.3.3.3 Neurodegenerative disease

By applying the Perturbing Regulatory Interactions by Synthetic Modulators (PRISM) to a yeast model of PD, sgRNAs were identified to modulate transcriptional networks and protect cells from α-Syn toxicity [38]. The APPswe (Swedish) mutation in the amyloid precursor protein (APP) gene causes Alzheimer's disease (AD). The mutant APP^{SW} allele can be selectively disrupted using CRISPRs/Cas9 both *ex vivo* and *in vivo* and thereby decrease pathogenic amyloid-β (Aβ) [39].

2.3.3.4 Cancer

CRISPRs/Cas9 were tried to inhibit hepatocellular carcinoma (HCC). miR-125b can suppress the expression of SIRT6 by directly targeting the seed-matching region of its 3′UTR. After the expression of *SIRT6* knocked out through CRISPRs/Cas9, HCC cells showed the decreased viability and invasiveness, which had the similar function upon the overexpression of the miR-125b [40]. CRISPRs/Cas9 was also tried to inhibit breast cancer. Cyclin-dependent kinases (CDKs) are established anti-cancer drug targets, and a new generation of CDK inhibitors provides clinical benefits to the patients. Breast cancer cells were genetically manipulated using a deactivated CRISPRs/Cas9 (dCRISPR) approach to strengthen the endogenous CDK18 promoter to express highly to exhibit an increased sensitivity [41].

3. Conclusion

The gene editing technologies, especially CRISPRs/Cas9, have been extensively used as tools in basic research for genome encoding, silencing, enhancing, and modification. Currently, they are further applied in manufacturing nonhuman therapeutic products and medicinal products. Particularly, the discovery of medicinal products using gene editing technologies will open a new era for human therapeutics and expect to bring a hope for patient recovery from being seriously sick. Many biotechnology companies and pharmaceutical plants have successfully produced products using gene editing technologies. For example, CRISPR has become an industry which is prosperously developing recently. Nonhuman therapeutic products are usually manufactured nonexclusively, while human therapeutic products are manufactured exclusively because they are highly technical, ethically concerned, and more profitable. Gene editing technologies are very promising in applications, though there are still many technical (e.g., off target effects, option of delivery tools, localization of function) and ethical challenges (e.g., evaluation of benefits and risks, compatibility of private interests and the public good, random manipulation of genes, commercialization of human therapy) unsolved. More and more products based on these technologies are approved for marketing. We also expect the challenges of safety concerns (e.g., genetically modified organism, tumorigenesis, etc.) and ethical issues will be overcome in the near future.

Author details

Yuan-Chuan Chen
Program in Comparative Biochemistry, University of California, Berkeley, CA, USA

*Address all correspondence to: yuchuan1022@gmail.com

References

[1] Im W, Moon J, Kim M. Applications of CRISPR/Cas9 for gene editing in hereditary movement disorders. Journal of Movement Disorders. 2016;**9**(3): 136-143. DOI: 10.14802/jmd.16029

[2] Urnov FD, Rebar EJ, Holmes MC, Zhang HS, Gregory PD. Genome editing with engineered zinc finger nucleases. Nature Reviews Genetics. 2010;**11**(9): 636-646. DOI: 10.1038/nrg2842

[3] Boch J, Scholze H, Schornack S, Landgraf A, Hahn S, Kay S, et al. Breaking the code of DNA binding specificity of TAL-type III effectors. Science. 2009;**326**(5959):1509-1512. DOI: 10.1126/science.1178811

[4] Li T, Huang S, Jiang WZ, Wright D, Spalding MH, Weeks DP, et al. TAL nucleases (TALNs): Hybrid proteins composed of TAL effectors and FokI DNA-cleavage domain. Nucleic Acids Research. 2011;**39**(1):359-372. DOI: 10.1093/nar/gkq704

[5] Wood AJ, Lo TW, Zeitler B, Pickle CS, Ralston EJ, Lee AH, et al. Targeted genome editing across species using ZFNs and TALEN. Science. 2011;**333**(6040):307. DOI: 10.1126/science.1207773

[6] Christian M et al. Targeting DNA double-strand breaks with TAL effector nucleases. Genetics. 2010;**186**(2): 757-761. DOI: 10.1534/genetics.110.120717

[7] Mussolino C, Morbitzer R, Lütge F, Dannemann N, Lahaye T, Cathomen T. A novel TALE nuclease scaffold enables high genome editing activity in combination with low toxicity. Nucleic Acids Research. 2011;**39**(21):9283-9293. DOI: 10.1093/nar/gkr597

[8] Hockemeyer D, Wang H, Kiani S, Lai CS, Gao Q, Cassady JP, et al. Genetic engineering of human pluripotent cells using TALE nucleases. Nature Biotechnology. 2011;**29**(8):731-734. DOI: 10.1038/nbt.1927

[9] Horvath P, Barrangou R. CRISPR/Cas, the immune system of bacteria and archaea. Science. 2010;**327**(5962):167-170. DOI: 10.1126/science

[10] DiCarlo JE, Norville JE, Mali P, Rios X, Aach J, Church GM. Genome engineering in *Saccharomyces cerevisiae* using CRISPR Cas systems. Nucleic Acids Research. 2013;**41**(7):4336-4343. DOI: 10.1093/nar/gkt135

[11] Charpentier E, Doudna JA. Biotechnology: Rewriting a genome. Nature. 2013;**495**(7439):50-51. DOI: 10.1038/495050a

[12] Sui T, Xu L, Lau YS, Liu D, Liu T, Gao Y, et al. Development of muscular dystrophy in a CRISPR-engineered mutant rabbit model with frame-disrupting ANO5 mutations. Cell Death and Disease. 2018;**9**(6):609. DOI: 10.1038/s41419-018-0674-y

[13] Yang J, Yi N, Zhang J, He W, He D, Wu W, et al. Generation and characterization of a hypothyroidism rat model with truncated thyroid stimulating hormone receptor. Scientific Reports. 2018;(1):4004. DOI: 10.1038/s41598-018-22405-7

[14] Maiti P, Manna J, Dunbar GL. Current understanding of the molecular mechanisms in Parkinson's disease: Targets for potential treatments. Translational Neurodegeneration. 2018;**6**:28. DOI: 10.1186/s40035-017-0099-z

[15] Makarova KS, Wolf YI, Koonin EV. The basic building blocks and evolution of CRISPR-CAS systems. Biochemical Society Transactions. 2013;**41**(6): 1392-1400. DOI: 10.1042/BST20130038

[16] Chen JS, Ma E, Harrington LB, Da Costa M, Tian X, Palefsky JM, et al. CRISPR-Cas12a target binding unleashes indiscriminate single-stranded DNase activity. Science. 2018;**360**(6387):436-439. DOI: 10.1126/science.aar6245

[17] Shi J, Wang E, Milazzo JP, Wang Z, Kinney JB, Vakoc CR. Discovery of cancer drug targets by CRISPR-Cas9 screening of protein domains. Nature Biotechnology. 2015;**33**(6):661-667. DOI: 10.1038/nbt.3235

[18] Liao Y, Bai Q, Xu P, Wu T, Guo D, Peng Y, et al. Mutation in rice *Abscisic Acid2* results in cell death, enhanced disease-resistance, altered seed dormancy and development. Frontiers in Plant Science. 2018;**9**:405. DOI: 10.3389/fpls.2018.00405

[19] Huang C, Sun H, Xu D, Chen Q, Liang Y, Wang X, et al. *ZmCCT9* enhances maize adaptation to higher latitudes. Proceedings of the National Academy of Sciences of the United States of America. 2018;**115**(2):E334-E341. DOI: 10.1073/pnas.1718058115

[20] Su X, Cui K, Du S, Li H, Lu F, Shi D, et al. Efficient genome editing in cultured cells and embryos of Debao pig and swamp buffalo using the CRISPR/Cas9 system. In Vitro Cellular & Developmental Biology Animal. 2018;**54**(5):375-383. DOI: 10.1007/s11626-018-0236-8

[21] Khalil K, Elayat M, Khalifa E, Daghash S, Elaswad A, Miller M, et al. Generation of myostatin gene-edited channel catfish (*Ictalurus punctatus*) via zygote injection of CRISPR/Cas9 system. Scientific Reports. 2018;**7**(1):7301. DOI: 10.1038/s41598-017-07223-7

[22] Barrangou R, Fremaux C, Deveau H, Richards M, Boyaval P, Romero DA, et al. CRISPR provides acquired resistance against viruses in prokaryotes. Science. 2007;**315**(5819):1709-1712. DOI: 10.1126/science.1138140

[23] Waltz E. Gene-edited CRISPR mushroom escapes US regulation. Nature. 2016;**532**(7599):293. DOI: 10.1038/nature.2016.19754

[24] Bozarth A, Maier UG, Zauner S. Diatoms in biotechnology: Modern tools and applications. Applied Microbiology and Biotechnology. 2009;**82**(2):195-201. DOI: 10.1007/s00253-008-1804-8

[25] Nymark M, Sharma AK, Sparstad T, Bones AM, Winge P. A CRISPR/Cas9 system adapted for gene editing in marine algae. Scientific Reports. 2016;**6**:24951. DOI: 10.1038/srep24951

[26] Shipman SL, Nivala J, Macklis JD, Church GM. CRISPR-Cas encoding of a digital movie into the genomes of a population of living bacteria. Nature. 2017;**547**(7663):345-349. DOI: 10.1038/nature23017

[27] Lynch VJ, Bedoya-Reina OC, Ratan A, Sulak M, Drautz-Moses DI, Perry GH, et al. Elephantid genomes reveal the molecular bases of woolly mammoth adaptations to the arctic. Cell Reports. 2015;**12**(2):217-228. DOI: 10.1016/j.celrep.2015.06.027

[28] Basu S, Adams L, Guhathakurta S, Kim YS. A novel tool for monitoring endogenous alpha-synuclein transcription by NanoLuciferase tag insertion at the 3′ end using CRISPR-Cas9 genome editing technique. Scientific Reports. 2017;**8**:45883. DOI: 10.1038/srep45883

[29] Deuse T, Hu X, Gravina A, Wang D, Tediashvili G, De C, et al. Hypoimmunogenic derivatives of induced pluripotent stem cells evade immune rejection in fully immunocompetent allogeneic

recipients. Nature Biotechnology. 2019;**37**(3):252-258. DOI: 10.1038/s41587-019-0016-3

[30] Perales MA, Kebriaei P, Kean LS, Sadelain M. Reprint of: Building a safer and faster CAR: Seatbelts, airbags, and CRISPR. Biology of Blood and Marrow Transplantation. 2018;**24**(3S):S15-S19. DOI: 10.1016/j.bbmt.2017.12.789

[31] van Diemen FR, Kruse EM, Hooykaas MJ, Bruggeling CE, Schürch AC, van Ham PM, et al. CRISPR/Cas9-mediated genome editing of herpesviruses limits productive and latent infections. PLoS Pathogens. 2016;**12**(6):e1005701. DOI: 10.1371/journal.ppat.1005701

[32] Imran M, Waheed Y, Ghazal A, Ullah S, Safi SZ, Jamal M, et al. Modern biotechnology-based therapeutic approaches against HIV infection. Biomedical Reports. 2017;**7**(6):504-507. DOI: 10.3892/br.2017.1006

[33] Yuen KS, Wang ZM, Wong NM, Zhang ZQ, Cheng TF, Lui WY, et al. Suppression of Epstein-Barr virus DNA load in latently infected nasopharyngeal carcinoma cells by CRISPR/Cas9. Virus Research. 2018;**244**:296-303. DOI: 10.1016/j.virusres.2017.04.019

[34] Lin SR, Yang HC, Kuo YT, Liu CJ, Yang TY, Sung KC, et al. The CRISPR/Cas9 system facilitates clearance of the intrahepatic HBV templates *in vivo*. Molecular Therapy--Nucleic Acids. 2014;**3**:e186. DOI: 10.1038/mtna.2014.38

[35] Chen J, Zhang W, Lin J, Wang F, Wu M, Chen C, et al. An efficient antiviral strategy for targeting hepatitis B virus genome using transcription activator-like effector nucleases. Molecular Therapy. 2014;**22**(2):303-311. DOI: 10.1038/mt.2013.212

[36] Noh KW, Park J, Kang MS. Targeted disruption of EBNA1 in EBV-infected cells attenuated cell growth. BMB Reports. 2016;**49**(4):226-231. DOI: 10.5483/BMBRep.2016.49.4.260

[37] Cohen J. The birth of CRISPR Inc. Science. 2017;**355**(6326):680-684. DOI: 10.1126/science.355.6326.680

[38] Chen YC, Farzadfard F, Gharaei N, Chen WCW, Cao J, Lu TK. Randomized CRISPR-Cas transcriptional perturbation screening reveals protective genes against alpha-synuclein toxicity. Molecular Cell. 2017;**68**(1):247.e5-257.e5. DOI: 10.1016/j.molcel.2017.09.014

[39] György B, Lööv C, Zaborowski MP, Takeda S, Kleinstiver BP, Commins C, et al. CRISPR/Cas9 mediated disruption of the Swedish APP allele as a therapeutic approach for early-onset Alzheimer's disease. Molecular Therapy--Nucleic Acids. 2018;**11**:429-440. DOI: 10.1016/j.omtn.2018.03.007

[40] Song S, Yang Y, Liu M, Liu B, Yang X, Yu M, et al. MiR-125b attenuates human hepatocellular carcinoma malignancy through targeting SIRT6. American Journal of Cancer Research. 2018;**8**(6):993-1007

[41] Barone G, Arora A, Ganesh A, Abdel-Fatah T, Moseley P, Ali R, et al. The relationship of CDK18 expression in breast cancer to clinicopathological parameters and therapeutic response. Oncotarget. 2018;**9**(50):29508-29524. DOI: 10.18632/oncotarget.25686

Section 2

Animal Research

Chapter 2

Application and Development of CRISPR/Cas9 Technology in Pig Research

Huafeng Lin, Qiudi Deng, Lili Li and Lei Shi

Abstract

Pigs provide valuable meat sources, disease models, and research materials for humans. However, traditional methods no longer meet the developing needs of pig production. More recently, advanced biotechnologies such as SCNT and genome editing are enabling researchers to manipulate genomic DNA molecules. Such methods have greatly promoted the advancement of pig research. Three gene editing platforms including ZFNs, TALENs, and CRISPR/Cas are becoming increasingly prevalent in life science research, with CRISPR/Cas9 now being the most widely used. CRISPR/Cas9, a part of the defense mechanism against viral infection, was discovered in prokaryotes and has now developed as a powerful and effective genome editing tool that can introduce and enhance modifications to the eukaryotic genomes in a range of animals including insects, amphibians, fish, and mammals in a predictable manner. Given its excellent characteristics that are superior to other tailored endonucleases systems, CRISPR/Cas9 is suitable for conducting pig-related studies. In this review, we briefly discuss the historical perspectives of CRISPR/Cas9 technology and highlight the applications and developments for using CRISPR/Cas9-based methods in pig research. We will also review the choices for delivering genome editing elements and the merits and drawbacks of utilizing the CRISPR/Cas9 technology for pig research, as well as the future prospects.

Keywords: applications, CRISPR/Cas9, delivery methods, gene editing, pig

1. Introduction

1.1 The status of pig production and current application of CRISPR/Cas9 technology

Worldwide, pig (*Sus scrofa domestica*) production accounted for 42% of total livestock production in 2018, and this percentage is expected to go up by the year 2050 [1, 2]. Pork, which makes up nearly 40% of all meat consumed by the world population, is clearly an important meat source for humans [3]. These production and consumption data reveal the significant implications of pigs for humans. Indeed, pigs bring many benefits for the convenience and survival of human beings. In light of the importance and necessity for pig production, researchers all around the world are using various methods to actively investigate this species.

Benefitting from the rapid development of genome-editing technologies during the last decade, many laboratories have applied this tool to animals, plants, and microorganisms in order to obtain both higher yield and better quality varieties. With the advent of the CRISPR (clustered regularly interspaced short palindromic repeats)/Cas9 technique and the melioration of delivery methods, gene editing can be more successfully performed in livestock such as swine. In addition, evidence shows that, in addition to primates, pigs share many similar characteristics with humans such as organ size, genome length, blood glucose levels, and the complexity and composition of chromosomes [4, 5], as well as the early embryonic development trajectory [6]. Therefore, pigs are not only used as important domestic animals for food and pharmaceutical applications, but also served as ideal animal models for simulating various human diseases (e.g., diabetes, obesity, and cardiovascular disease). In this manuscript, we first introduce the historical perspectives of gene-editing technologies in pigs, review the latest advances in the utilization of CRISPR/Cas9 strategies for swine research, and then describe possible methods for delivering these genome-editing components, as well as the future perspective on pig studies by using this technology.

1.2 Historical background of gene editing in pigs

CRISPR, discovered in 1987, is a family of DNA sequences of short direct repeats interspaced with short sequences. Its mechanism of action has been confirmed to be related with acquired immunity of microbes [7–9]. By 2000, researchers had discovered that these specific sequences occurred in about 40% of bacteria and 90% of archaea [10, 11]. In 2002, this interesting architecture, initially named short regularly spaced repeats (SRSRs), was renamed as the clustered regularly interspaced short palindromic repeats (CRISPRs) [10, 12]. Between 2002 and 2009, a series of proteins associated with these palindromic sequences were identified as constituents of the complicated mechanism of microbial adaptive immunity [11]. In 2014, the X-ray crystal structure of *Streptococcus pyogenes* Cas9 (*Sp*Cas9) in complex with sgRNA was elucidated [13, 14]. Nowadays, *Sp*Cas9 endonuclease, which requires a protospacer adjacent motif (PAM) sequence (5'-NGG-3′), is routinely designed as a 'molecular scissor' guided by a single guide RNA (or dual-tracrRNA) due to simple structural characteristics, the advantages of easy operation, and high efficiency [11, 15]. Notably, the multiplex abilities of the Cas9-associated guided RNAs (gRNAs) and the diverse Cas9 orthologs (e.g., *Sp*Cas9, *Sa*Cas9, *St*Cas9) as well as the diversified Cas9 variants (**Figure 1**) have enabled CRISPR/Cas9 systems to be used in a wide range of research applications [16, 17].

As early as 1985, the first transgenic pig was created by direct DNA microinjection of the metallothionein-I/human growth hormone (MT/hGH) fusion gene into a fertilized egg [18]. Further technical enhancements occurred during the next 20 years, until, in 2011, Whitworth and his co-workers were the first to successfully apply ZFN technology to generate cloned eGFP knockout pigs [19]. Similarly, Carlson et al. (2012) pioneered the application of TALENs in editing the porcine genome, and they produced low-density lipoprotein receptor (LDLR) knockout pigs [20]. By 2013, the groundbreaking work of genome engineering in mammalian cells based on the CRISPR/Cas9 system had been achieved [21]. The first examples of genome-modified pigs engineered using the CRISPR/Cas9 technique were reported almost simultaneously by Hai et al. (2014) [22] and Whitworth et al. (2014) [23]. From then on, rapid and efficient CRISPR/Cas9-mediated genome editing in pigs has opened up many more possibilities for applications in biology and biomedicine.

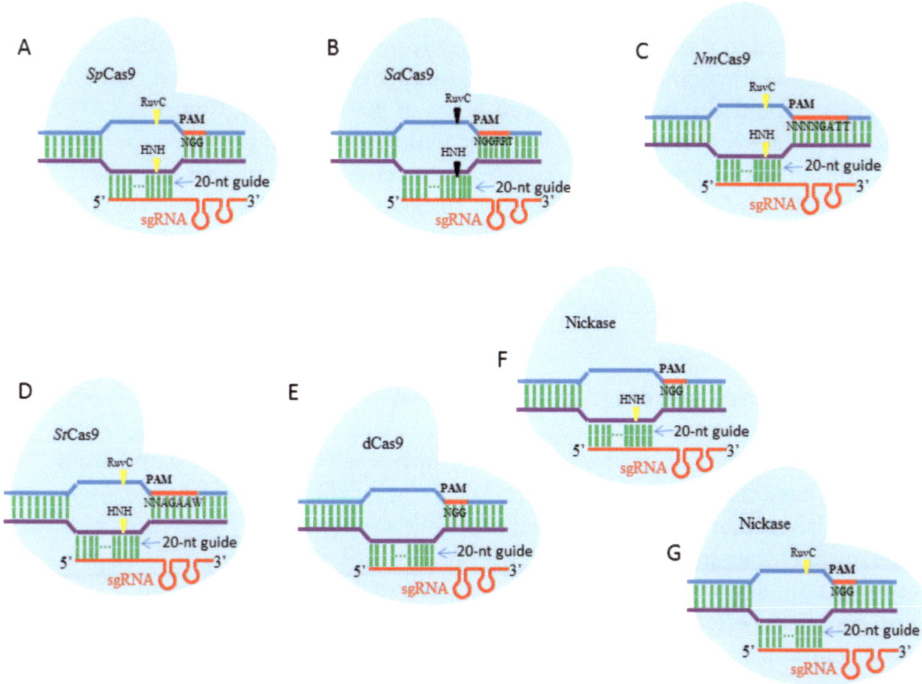

Figure 1.
Diagram illustrating different types of engineered CRISPR/Cas9 and its Cas9 variants. (A) The wild-type SpCas9 nuclease. (B) The wild-type SaCas9 nuclease. (C) The wild-type NmCas9 nuclease. (D) The wild-type StCas9 nuclease. (E) The dCas9 variant can bind DNA but cannot cut DNA strands. (F) The SpCas9 nickase that can only introduce a single strand break at the HNH nuclease domain. (G) The SpCas9 nickase that can only introduce a single strand break at the RuvC nuclease domain. (SpCas9, Streptococcus pyogenes Cas9; SaCas9, Staphylococcus aureus Cas9; NmCas9, Neisseria meningitides Cas9; StCas9, Streptococcus thermophilus Cas9; dCas9, catalytically inactive ("dead") Cas9; sgRNA, single-guide RNA; PAM, protospacer adjacent motif; W = A or T). Refer to [16].

2. Application and development

2.1 Applications in the antimicrobial and antiviral fields

Currently, the traditional methods for developing pig anti-viral vaccines are time-consuming and labor-intensive [24]. Cas9 endonucleases, as molecular DNA scissors guided by gRNA, are now used to target and cut exogenous DNA arising from virus or plasmids [25]. With the development of state-of-the-art biotechnologies, scientists now can utilize this revolutional tool to prevent domestic pigs from pathogenic bacterial and viral attack. In 2016, Liang and his colleagues developed a rapid vaccine development method based on the combination of CRISPR/Cas9 and the Cre/Lox system to fight against the re-emerging pseudorabies virus (PRV). The results demonstrated the protective efficacy of this candidate vaccine in swine and showed promise in controlling the outbreak of pseudorabies [26]. In another trial, Whitworth et al. (2015) employed the CRISPR/Cas9 system to directionally mutate the CD163 gene (cluster of differentiation 163 gene, a gate keeper gene associated with PRRSV) in order to create biallelic gene knockout pigs which had protective immunity against infection of porcine reproductive and respiratory syndrome virus (PRRSV) [27]. In 2018, Xie and his co-workers applied the combinational method of CRISPR/Cas9 and RNAi to generate anti-CSFV transgenic pigs and confirmed that these pigs could impede the multiplication of classical swine fever virus (CSFV). They further proved that the disease resistance traits presented in the transgenic sows could be stably transmitted to their F1-generation offspring. This study suggested that the use of such transgenic pigs would offer potential benefits over commercial vaccination, could substantially reduce CSFV-related economic losses, and would also improve the well-being of livestock [28]. Compared to CSFV, African swine fever virus (ASFV) is a very acute, lethal viral pathogen for both domestic and wild pigs, but unfortunately, a vaccine candidate that effectively prevents ASFV infection remains elusive. HüBner et al. (2018) applied the CRISPR/Cas9 nuclease system to target the double-stranded DNA genome of ASFV. In vitro culture experiments showed that mediated targeting of the ASFV p30 gene using this system is a feasible strategy to fight against ASFV infection, and may also be applied to the natural animal host [29].

2.2 Applications to breeding and reproduction

Traditional breeding methods, which comprise selective breeding and cross-breeding, have clearly hit a bottleneck. Additionally, due to the long time, high cost, and high labor intensity of traditional breeding methods [30], researchers now hope to find other alternatives that are more convenient and efficient than previously. Genome-editing technology can help us to achieve a good result in a short time, and help better understand swine reproduction. Interestingly, many aspects of pig reproduction are suitable as translational models of reproduction in humans, including oocyte maturation, sperm-egg interaction mechanism, tubo-uterine contractility, early embryo development, pregnancy, fetal genome modification, and reproductive diseases [31]. Strategies that use the CRISPR/Cas9 technique to improve the reproduction in swine are becoming more prevalent. PRRSV, a virus associated with reproductive and respiratory disease, can cause severe unsuccessful reproductive outcomes in sows, decrease sperm quality in infected boars, and lower the birth rates of healthy piglets [32]. In 2016, Tao et al. generated efficient biallelic mutation in porcine parthenotes by cytoplasmic injection of Cas9/sgRNA mixtures. These data emphasize the function of parthenotes in revealing early embryonic development and assessing mutation efficiency [33]. In the same year, Whitworth et al. used CRISPR/Cas9 to generate CD163-knockout pigs to protect pig from PRRSV and reduce the incidence of reproductive disease, important for pig studies in both the fields of reproduction and anti-viruses [27]. In 2017, Park et al. utilized CRISPR/Cas9 technology to program the NANOS2 gene in domestic pigs to generate offspring with monoallelic and biallelic mutations. They found that NANOS2 knockout pigs presented the phenotype of male specific germ line ablation but other aspects of testicular development were normal. The exception was male pigs with one intact NANOS2 allele and female knockout pigs which both maintained good reproductive performance [34].

2.3 Applications in immunization and xenotransplantation

Swines, having many highly similar anatomical and physiological features to humans, are considered to be the excellent donors for patients in the case of a shortage of human organs for allogenic transplantation [35, 36]. However, several issues still need to be addressed such as hyperacute rejection which can develop in recipients within several minutes after organ xenotransplantations [36, 37]. The advancement of the CRISPR/Cas9 technique has greatly strengthened the ability to effectively manipulate porcine genome in order to evaluate and generate porcine organs that can assist in xenotransplantation.

An early study, undertaken by Sato and his research team in 2013, used a modified CRISPR/Cas9 system to knockout the porcine GGTA1 gene, whose protein product is responsible for the biosynthesis of the a-Gal epitope, which leads to hyperacute rejection upon pig-to-human xenotransplantation. This trial not only demonstrated that CRISPR/Cas9 is a promising tool for producing knockout cloned piglets, but also paved the way for pig-to-human xenotransplantation [38]. Piglets with biallelic knockouts of GGTA1 gene were eventually created by Petersen and his colleagues [39] using the combined technologies of CRISPR/Cas9 and somatic cell nuclear transfer (SCNT).

Swine could also serve as an ideal animal model for investigating viral immunity and immune rejection in xenotransplantation if they are deficient in class I MHC. Research published by Reyes et al. in 2014 utilized the Cas9 endonuclease with chimeric gRNAs to generate class I MHC knockout piglets as promising experimental animals for immunological research [40]. In 2015, Yang and co-workers designed two Cas9 gRNA molecules to inactivate 62 copies of the pol gene required for porcine endogenous retrovirus (PERV) activity. This study performed on porcine kidney epithelial cell lines demonstrated that the modifications could greatly reduce in vitro spreading of PERVs to human cells, raising the hope of the eradication of such viruses from pigs for heterograft donors [41]. One year later, Yang's research team (2017) made further progress in employing CRISPR/Cas9 technology to inactivate all the PERVs in a porcine primary cell line and produced PERV-eliminated pigs using the SCNT technique. The experimental results addressed the safety problem in clinical xenotransplantation due to the success of impeding interspecific transmission of viruses [42].

2.4 Disease models and translational medical research

The CRISPR/Cas9 technology has both simplified and expedited biomedical modeling for some refractory human diseases. One way to combat human diseases is to create genetically modified animal models for investigating the mechanism of diseases enabling the development of safe and effective drugs. An effective animal disease model should appropriately simulate the *in vivo* environment under investigation and respond or react to stimuli in a similar manner to the human body [43–45]. Commonly used animal models in the laboratory include mice, rats, dogs, monkey, and swine. The pig models have been developed to faithfully mimic various human diseases including neurodegenerative diseases [46], cancers [45], and gastrointestinal (GI) tract diseases [47] as they share similar features to humans in terms of anatomy, physiology, and genetics [43]. Gene editing using CRISPR/Cas9 technology is proving an innovative and effective research tool, which is greatly revolutionizing our ability to manipulate the porcine genome to create appropriate disease models.

As early as 2013, Tan et al. used two custom endonucleases (TALEN and CRISPR/Cas9 system) to edit azoospermia-like (DAZL) and adenomatous polyposis coli (APC) loci in the pig genome. The results suggested that gene editing could be incorporated into selection programs to accelerate genetic improvement, with applications in animal breeding and human personalized medicine [48]. In 2014, Zhou et al. were the first to report that zygote injection of a customized CRISPR/Cas9 system could efficiently generate genome-modified pigs (biallelic knockout pigs) in one step, which provided an important animal model for the treatment of human type I and III *von* Willebrand disease [22]. At the end of 2015, Peng et al. adopted the CRISPR/Cas9 method to knockin human cDNA into the albumin gene locus in pig zygotes and successfully produced human albumin from porcine blood [49]. Additionally, Feng et al. (2015) reported the potential of using the combination of CRISPR/Cas9 and human pluripotent stem cells (PSCs) to harvest human organs from chimeric swine [50]. In 2016, Wang et al. performed a study in which Cas9 mRNA and multiple single guide RNAs (sgRNAs), which respectively specifically target to parkin, DJ-1, and PINK1 gene loci, were coinjected into in vivo derived pronuclear embryos of Bama miniature pigs. There were only minor low off-target events. These results demonstrated the capability of using the CRISPR/Cas9 system to trigger genetic modification of multiple sites in pigs, yielding positive results with high medical value [51]. In the same year, Lee and his team utilized genome-specific CRISPR/Cas9 systems to target runt-related transcription factor 3 (RUNX3, a known tumor suppressor gene) to generate a pig model that can recapitulate the pathogenesis of RUNX3-associated stomach cancer in humans. The results demonstrated that the CRISPR/Cas9 system was effective in inducing mutations on a specific locus of the pig genome, resulting in the generation of piglets lacking RUNX3 protein in their internal organs. This system brings useful resources (RUNX3 knockout pigs) for human cancer research and the development of novel cancer therapies [52]. In 2017, Zhang et al. designed an experiment that applied the CRISPR/Cas9 system and SCNT technology to generate complement protein C3 targeted piglets, which could be a valuable large animal model for elucidating the roles of C3, a protein of the immune system that plays a central role in the complement system and contributes to innate immunity [53]. By 2018, following many years' efforts, scientists have now made significant progress in using CRISPR/Cas9-mediated knockin techniques to produce a Huntington's disease (HD) pig model, which assists in the investigation of the pathogenesis of neurodegenerative diseases and the development of appropriate therapeutics [54]. Recently (2018), Cho and co-workers successfully used the CRISPR/Cas9 and SCNT technologies to generate INS knockout pigs (insulin-deficient pigs) and demonstrated the efficacy of the CRISPR/Cas9 system in producing pig models for use in diabetes research and pharmaceutical testing [55].

2.5 Improvement of meat quality and food safety

Pig meat quality is controlled by multiple factors. To some extent, genetics are considered as the dominating factor influencing pork quality in the pig industry, although environmental conditions can also potentially influence the porcine genetics in the long term. In addition, fat and lean meat contents are both important for the palatability of the pork [56, 57] and diet considerations. Consequently, scientists now propose to improve pork traits to cater for the taste of the general public by using gene-editing technology. In 2016, Bi et al. constructed isozygous, functional myostatin (MSTN) knockout cloned pigs without selectable marker gene (SMG) by combined use of CRISPR/Cas9 and Cre/LoxP. The results showed that compared to the control group, the skeleton muscles were more pronounced and the back fat thickness decreased slightly in such gene-edited pigs [58]. In 2017, Zheng et al. established a CRISPR/Cas9-mediated homologous recombination-independent approach to efficiently insert mouse adiponectin-UCP1 into the porcine endogenous uncoupling protein 1 (UCP1) locus. The resultant UCP1 knockin pigs showed an enhanced ability to control their body temperature during acute cold exposure, lower fat deposition, and increased carcass lean meat [59]. In 2018, Xiang et al. used CRISPR/Cas9 technology to effectively edit insulin-like growth factor 2 (IGF2) intron 3–3072 site as the method of choice for the improvement of meat production in Bama pigs. The result showed that it was the first time to demonstrate that editing a noncoding region can ameliorate economic traits in livestock [60].

CRISPR/Cas9 gene-editing technology has multiple benefits. In gene detection fields, Zhou et al. developed a CRISPR/Cas9-triggered nicking endonuclease-mediated strand displacement amplification method (namely CRISDA) for amplifying and detecting double-stranded DNA [61]. CRISDA promises to be a

Authors/year/refs	Cells/organisms	Genomic loci	CRISPR/ Cas9 delivery platforms	Gene-editing modes	CRISPR/Cas9 formats	Comments/results
Hai et al., 2014, [22]	Zygote	*v*WF	Cytoplasmic injection	Knockout	Cas9 mRNA and sgRNA	Constructed pig disease modes using CRISPR/Cas9
Sato et al., 2014, [38]	PEFs	GGTA1	Plasmids/ transfection	Knockout/ CNT	CRISPR/Cas9 plasmids DNA and sgRNA	Efficiently mutated portion of GGTA1
Whitworth et al., 2014, [23]	PFF cells	eGFP/CD163/CD1D	Plasmids/ transfection/ microinjection	Knockout	Cas9 plasmids DNA and sgRNA	Generated GE pigs for mutating two genes
Chen et al., 2015, [68]	PFFs	J_H	Plasmids/ transfection/ electroporation	Knockout/ SCNT	Cas9-sgRNA plasmids	Generated a B cell-deficient phenotype in pig
Li et al., 2015, [69]	Liver-derived cells	GGTA1/CMAH/ iGB3S	Plasmids/ transfection	Knockout/ SCNT	Cas9 plasmids and multiplexed sgRNA	Modified multiple genetic in a single pregnancy
Peng et al., 2015, [49]	Zygotes	Alb	Microinjection	Knockin	Cas9 mRNA and sgRNA	Knockined Alb gene and produced albumin in the blood of piglets
Ruan et al., 2015, [63]	PFFs	pH11	Plasmids/ electroporation	Knockin	Cas9/sgRNA targeting plasmids	Inserted foreign gene into the pH11 locus
Wang et al., 2015, [70]	Oocytes/PPFs	MITF	Microinjection	Knockout/ knockin	Cas9 mRNA and sgRNA	Expanded the practical possibilities in pigs
Zhou et al., 2015, [64]	PFFs	TYR/PARK2 /PINK1	Plasmids/ transfection	Knockout/ SCNT	Cas9 plasmids and sgRNA	Gene-targeted pigs can be effectively achieved
Kang et al., 2016, [52]	PFFs	RUNX3	Plasmids/ transfection/ electroporation	Knockout	Cas9-sgRNA plasmids	Generated pig disease mode for cancer research
Petersen et al., 2016, [39]	Oocytes	GGTA1	Intracytoplasmic microinjection	Knockout	(Cas9 and sgRNA) expression DNA	GGTA1 knockout pigs could bring xenotransplantation closer to clinical application

Authors/year/refs	Cells/organisms	Genomic loci	CRISPR/ Cas9 delivery platforms	Gene-editing modes	CRISPR/Cas9 formats	Comments/results
Wang et al., 2016, [51]	Zygotes	parkin/DJ-1/PINK1	Co-injection	Knockout	Cas9 mRNA and multiplexing sgRNAs	Modified multiple genes in pigs
Yang et al., 2016, [65]	PFFs	pINS	Plasmids/ electroporation	SCNT	Cas9 plasmids/sgRNA	Generated the genetically modified pigs exclusively expressing human insulin
Yu et al., 2016, [73]	Zygotes	DMD	Plasmids/ microinjection	Knockout	Cas9 mRNA and sgRNA	Targeted of DMD gene in miniature pig
Chuang et al., 2017, [71]	Fertilized eggs	GGTA1	Plasmids/ microinjection	Knockout	CRISPR/Cas9 plasmids DNA	Firstly used porcine U6 promoter to express gRNA to generate GGTA1 mutant pigs with PBMCs
Gao et al., 2017, [74]	PFFs	GGTA1/CMAH	Plasmids/ handmade cloning (HMC)	Knockout	Cas9-coding DNA and sgRNA	Modified multiple genes in pigs
Huang et al., 2017, [75]	PEFs	ApoE/LDLR	Plasmids/ electroporation	Knockout/ SCNT	(Cas9 and sgRNA) expression DNA	Generated genetically modified pigs targeting the ApoE and LDLR genes simultaneously
Li et al., 2017, [76]	Oocytes/PFFs	TPH2	Plasmids/ electroporation	Knockout/ SCNT	(Cas9 and sgRNA) expression DNA	Tph2 targeted piglets were successfully generated
Park et al., 2017, [34]	Oocytes	NANOS2	Plasmids	Knockout	Cas9:GFP mRNA and sgRNA	Edited the NANOS2 gene to generate germline ablated male pigs
Whitworth et al., 2017, [72]	Zygote	TMRPSS2	Plasmids/ microinjection	Mutation	sgRNA and Cas9 mRNA	Successfully modified the target gene
Wu et al., 2017, [77]	Oocytes	PDX1	Microinjection	Knockin	Cas9 mRNA and dual sgRNAs	Xeno-generated of human tissues and organs in pigs
Zheng et al., 2017, [59]	FFAs	UCP1	Plasmids	Knockin	Cas9-sgRNA plasmids	Improves pig welfare and reduces economic losses
Borca et al., 2018, [78]	Primary swine macrophage	8-DR	Plasmids	Targeted deletion	Cas9 plasmids/sgRNA	Used CRISPR-Cas9 system to produce recombinant ASFVs

Authors/year/refs	Cells/organisms	Genomic loci	CRISPR/Cas9 delivery platforms	Gene-editing modes	CRISPR/Cas9 formats	Comments/results
Cho et al., 2018, [55]	Porcine primary fibroblasts	INS	Plasmids/electroporation	Knockout	Cas9:GFP mRNA and sgRNA	Demonstrated effectiveness of CRISPR/Cas9 in generating new pig models
Hübner et al., 2018, [29]	ASFV-permissive WSL cells	CP204L	Plasmids	Targeted deletion	(Cas9 and sgRNA) expression DNA	CRISPR/Cas9 mediated targeting of the ASFV p30 gene is a valid strategy to convey resistance against ASF infection
Santos et al., 2018, [79]	Pig aortic endothelial cells	pTHBD	Plasmids	Knockout/recombination	(Cas9 and sgRNA) expression DNA	Create pigs with human genes in orthotopic position (hTHBD was inserted into the pTHBD locus)
Sato et al., 2018, [80]	zygote	GGTA1	Microinjection	Knockout	Cas9 mRNA and sgRNA; plasmid encoding humanized Cas9 and sgRNA	Developing a technique that reduces mosaicism is a key factor for production of knockout pigs
Xie et al., 2018, [28]	Porcine kidney cell/PFFs	Porcine ROSA26	Plasmids/electroporation	Knockin/SCNT	(Cas9 and sgRNA) expression DNA	Successfully produced anti-CSFV pigs
Yan et al., 2018, [54]	PFFs	HTT	Plasmids/electroporation	Knockout/SCNT	(Cas9 and sgRNA) expression DNA	First time to produce HD pig models for investigating the pathogenesis of neurodegenerative diseases
Yang et al., 2018, [81]	PFFs	CD163	Plasmids/electroporation	Knockout/SCNT	(Cas9 and sgRNA) expression plasmids	Demonstrated that CD163 knockout confers full resistance to HP-PRRSV infection to pigs

Acronyms and abbreviations: apolipoprotein E (ApoE); albumin (Alb); cysteine-rich domain 163 (CD163); CMP-Neu5Ac Hydroxylase (CMAH); duchenne muscle dystrophy (DMD); huntingtin (HTT); insulin (INS); microphthalmia-associated transcription factor (MITF); pancreatic duodenal homeobox-1 (PDX-1); porcine aortic endothelial cells (pAECs); porcine fetal fibroblasts (PFFs); pig embryonic fibroblast cells (PEFs); PTEN-induced kinase 1 (PINK1); Huntington's disease (HD); runt-related transcription factor 3 (RUNX3); thrombomodulin (THBD); tryptophan hydroxylase 2 (TPH2); transmembrane protease, serine 2 (TMPRSS2); tyrosinase (TYR); von Willebrand factor (vWF); wild boar lung (WSL).

Table 1. *Examples for the applications of CRISPR/Cas9 technology in pigs.*

powerful isothermal tool for ultrasensitive and specific detection of nucleic acids in pig pathogeny detection and food safety. Consequently, by making good use of this precision editing engineered technology in agriculture, a reliable avenue for elite swine production could be guaranteed, potential biological risks can be minimized, and a higher food safety can be protected.

2.6 Applications in transgenesis and beyond

Pig transgenesis is an important facet for functional investigation of biological pathways, as well as for biotechnology in animal husbandry. As a promising tool, CRISPR/Cas9 now has the ability to accelerate the process of pig transgenesis. Several studies have successfully constructed a CRISPR/Cas9 system for targeting the pig GGTA1 gene [38, 39, 62]. Ruan et al. (2015) inserted a gene fragment larger than 9 kb at the newly named pH 11 genomic locus using CRISPR/Cas9 technology and then confirmed that it was highly expressed in cells, embryos, and animals [63]. Similarly, Zhou et al. (2015) worked on CRISPR/Cas9-mediated gene targeting in porcine fetal fibroblasts (PFFs), in which TYR, PARK2, and PINK1 loci were effectively edited [64]. In 2016, Yang and colleagues edited the porcine INS (pINS) gene in fibroblasts by using TALENs or CRISPR/Cas9 [65], and in 2017, Zheng et al. inserted a mouse adiponectin-UCP1 gene efficiently into the porcine endogenous UCP1 locus by the utilization of a CRISPR/Cas9-mediated homologous recombination-independent approach [59]. In the same year, Wang et al. applied the combined system of Cre recombinase and Cas9/sgRNAs to simultaneously inactivate five tumor suppressor genes (TP53, PTEN, APC, BRCA1, and BRCA2) and activate one oncogene (KRAS) to develop a rapid lung tumor model in pigs [66]. By 2018, Whitworth et al. had developed a method that utilized the CRISPR/Cas9 technology to remove a loxP flanked neomycin cassette by direct zygote injection of RNA encoding Cre recombinase. This new technique can be used to efficiently remove selectable markers in genetically engineered animals without the need for long-term cell culture and subsequent somatic cell nuclear transfer (SCNT) [67]. Almost certainly, it has a very promising future for transgenic pigs with the advantages of enhancing body growth and minimizing environmental pollution that would be created by the CRISRP/Cas9 method. **Table 1** shows applications of CRISRP/Cas9 technology in transgenic pigs.

3. Delivery methods of CRISPR/Cas9

3.1 The appropriate choices for delivery: viral systems or nonviral platforms?

In order to introduce precise and efficient genome modification, the proper delivery modalities of CRISPR/Cas9 genome-editing materials are a crucial factor in the generation of genetically engineered pigs. A variety of strategies have been used for delivering the CRISPR/Cas9 system which can be mainly divided into viral and nonviral delivery methods (**Figure 2**) [82].

Viral systems are the traditional tools that have been widely used for delivering genome editing materials (DNA or mRNA). To-date, three viral vectors including lentivirus [83], adenovirus, and adeno-associated virus (AAV) have been used for delivery of CRISPR/Cas9 components in various biological studies [84, 85]. However, there are several limitations associated with viral vectors including immunogenicity, packaging capacity, broad tropism, and difficulty in production.

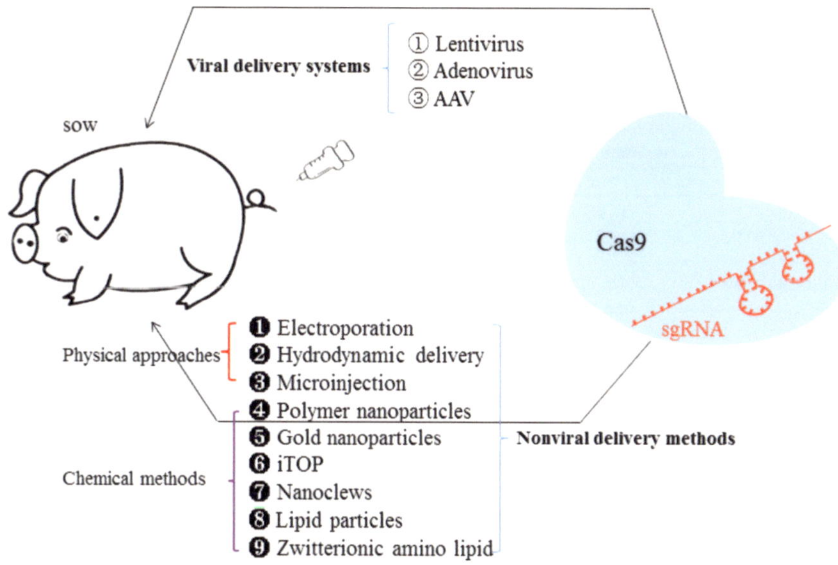

Figure 2.
Delivery techniques for the CRISPR/Cas9 system. (iTOP: induced transduction by osmocytosis and propanebetaine; AAV: adeno-associated virus).

Nonviral platforms for transferring the CRISPR/Cas9 components can be achieved by physical and chemical approaches. In contrast to viral vectors, non-viral vectors have lower immunogenicity, are not constrained by packaging sizes, are facile to synthesize, and are capable of carrying multiple sgRNAs simultaneously [86, 87]. In nonviral methods, genome editing reagents are delivered either as mRNA or as a combination of Cas9 endonuclease and sgRNA. To date, nonviral methods available include microinjection, electroporation [88], hydrodynamic injection, lipid particles, nanoclews, zwitterionic amino lipid (ZAL) nanoparticles, and iTOP as well as the combinations of viral and nonviral methods [82]. Herein, we compared the various methods for delivering the CRISRP/Cas9 system (**Table 2**).

Delivery methods of gene modification in the field of pig research have even used sperms as vectors for foreign genes (*e.g.* sperm-mediated gene transfer (SMGT), and intracytoplasmic sperm injection (ICSI)-mediated gene transfer), and delivery strategies such as retroviruses and lentiviruses are still current [100]. Somatic cell nuclear transfer (SCNT), a technique that consists of taking an enucleated oocyte and then implanting a donor nucleus from a somatic cell, is a remarkable breakthrough in the history of swine genetic engineering [101, 102]. SCNT combined with the rapid development of gene editing technologies such as TALENs and CRISPR/Cas9 has excellent prospects.

3.2 Challenges for delivering the CRISPR/Cas9 systems

The CRISPR/Cas9 system has been applied to genome modification in a variety of microorganisms, plants, and animals (including pigs), but the efficient transfer of such system is still a challenge that affects the precise genome-editing activity [103]. If the CRISPR/Cas9 systems are to effectively function in the targeted cells or organisms, choosing a suitable delivery system is of critical importance. According to existing research, the CRISPR/Cas9 system can be broadly divided into three kinds of packaging formats: Cas9 protein and sgRNA, Cas9 mRNA and

Delivery modes	Advantages	Limitations	Text refs
Lentivirus	Broad cell tropism; large capacity; long-term gene expression	Prone to insertional mutagenesis; transgene silencing; potential in carcinogenesis	[84], [89], [87], [90]
Adenovirus	High efficiency and versatility	Difficult to manufacture in scale; immunogenicity	[84], [91]
Adeno-associated virus	Minimal immunogenicity; non-pathogenic	Limited packaging size; potential to cause significant genomic damage	[14], [92], [93]
Electroporation	High transfection efficiency; suitable for all types of CRISPR-Cas9	Cytotoxicity; difficult for *in vivo* use	[94], [95]
Hydrodynamic delivery	Virus-free; easy-to-use; low-cost	Non-specific; tissue-invasive	[89], [96], [97]
Microinjection	Highly specific and reproducible	Time-consuming; suitable for *in vitro* applications; low-throughput	[94], [87]
Polymer nanoparticles	Safe; low-cost; simple manipulation; greater encapsulation capability	Low delivery efficiency	[94], [92]
Gold nanoparticles	Membrane-fusion-like delivery	Nonspecific inflammatory response; potential toxicity	[89], [98]
iTOP	Use for the delivery of Cas9 protein and sgRNA	Need to master sophisticated operating skills	[84], [89]
Nanoclews	Virus-free	Need to modify the template DNA	[99]

Table 2.
Comparison of different delivery methods for CRISPR/Cas9 system.

sgRNA, and CRISPR/Cas9 plasmid. Different CRISPR/Cas9 formats cooperate with special transport vehicle to complete the transportation task for gene-editing elements. Some research studies indicate that CRISPR/Cas9 ribonucleoprotein (RNP) delivery seems to exceed gene delivery as it provides multiple function advantages: short-term delivery, no insertional mutagenesis, minimal immunogenicity, and low off-target effect [87]. As previously mentioned, viral vectors usually have their own limitations to be overcome compared to nonviral vectors. However, nonviral vectors are generally used for *in vitro* genome editing studies due to their biological incompatibility or cytotoxicity [95]. Recently, developing efficient and biocompatible nonviral vectors (e.g., liposome and nanocarrier) has just emerged, and achievements have been made. For example, a low cytotoxic cationic polymer has been proven to mediate efficient CRISPR/Cas9 plasmid delivery for genome editing [92]. In addition, a research article presented that lipid-based Cas9 mRNA delivery has lower off-target effects than lentivirus-packaged Cas9 mRNA transportation [104]. Generally speaking, the packaging modes and delivery tools are two biggest factors that affect efficiency of the CRISPR/Cas9 system apart from this system itself. In order to describe the possible challenges for delivering the CRISPR/Cas9 system and the strategies used to overcome these challenges, we form a table to illustrate in detail (**Table 3**) and further to promote much research applications appropriately.

Challenges	Delivery methods	Strategies	Text refs
Off-target effects	Both in viral and nonviral vectors; using plasmid-based system	Engineering high specificity Cas9 protein; optimizing sgRNA design; proper selection of targeting site	[105], [94]
Packaging challenges	AAV (~4.7kpb), adenovirus, lentivirus (~10kpb)	Nonviral vectors have no packaging limitation, easy to prepare, and low in cost	[87], [106]
Insertional mutagenesis	AAV, adenovirus, lentivirus, retrovirus	Using Cas9–RNP for delivering; improved specificity	[87], [93], [107]
Mosaic genotypes	Microinjection	Stimulating the HDR pathway; use of Cas9 nickase	[108]
Immunogenicity	AAV, adenovirus, lentivirus, retrovirus	Using nonviral vectors to lower immunogenicity	[87], [95], [109]
Editing efficiency (transfection efficiency)	Nonviral vectors (not including electroporation)	Need to be further optimized; combination of viral vectors and nonviral vectors	[16], [95]
Systemic delivery	Viral and nonviral vectors	Difficult to achieve through nonviral vectors; tailoring new carriers	[16], [87]
Targeted delivery	Nonviral vectors	Viral vectors provide tissue tropism	[110]

Table 3.
Challenges for delivering the CRISPR/Cas9 system and the strategies that respond to these challenges.

4. Discussion

CRISPR/Cas9 technology is not only simple and easy to perform, but also has significantly improved performances for mutational studies, which has accelerated the application of the CRISPR/Cas9 toolkit [68, 111]. However, there are still some limitations and difficulties in the use of the CRISPR/Cas9 system for pig research.

1. The CRISPR/Cas9 system itself is not flawless, and its off-site concerns vary in different biological species [112, 113]. In addition, if the design and construction of sgRNA are not ideal, off-target editing of the genomic DNA can easily occur. With more available datasets of CRISPR/Cas9, more newfangled tools for designing sgRNA will be developed to lower the off-target effects.

2. In pigs, complex traits associated with multiple genes enhance the difficulties of using CRISPR/Cas9 to simultaneously and precisely edit and program DNA in the porcine genome.

3. Complex environmental factors including water sources and feed qualities, as well as animal husbandry production methods, as a range of external stimuli, could collaboratively affect CRISPR/Cas9-derived pigs in the long-term.

4. Strategies and timing for delivering CRISPR/Cas9 systems need to be optimized to control the ratio of HDR to NHEJ in order to enhance the efficiency of homology-directed recombination (HDR)-mediated precise gene modification [105].

5. Cytotoxicity produced by the CRISPR/Cas_9 system and toxic response to CRISPR/Cas_9 in mammalian cells has become an issue that must be taken into account. Recently, there have been reports that DSBs induced by Cas_9 triggered a P53-dependent toxic response that reduced the editing efficiency when applying the CRISPR/Cas_9 system to human programmed cells [114, 115]. Corresponding studies on pigs have not yet been undertaken, but the human studies provide some useful lessons for the development of pig research on genome editing.

6. Using the resulting fetuses or newborns edited by CRISPR/Cas_9 for screening of effective clones is time-consuming and laborious [80]. Probably, the method of T7E1 assay for detecting insertion/deletion (INDEL) mutations in blastocysts could help researchers to save time and money [80].

5. Conclusion

Over the past few years, genome-editing technology clearly allows scientists to produce genetically engineered pigs that are healthier to consume and more resistant to diseases in an efficient way. Nowadays, the use of the CRISPR/Ca9 technique on pigs in immunity, autoimmunity, obesity, aging, etc. is increasingly expanding and showing advantages over the conventional methods. In addition, another version of CRISPR named CRISPR/Cpf1 was discovered in microbes, which further expanded the CISPR toolkit, and holds promise to be applied in pig research. CRISPR/Ca9-modified pigs are providing a better perspective for understanding various aspects of pig biology and are paving the way for advancing the fields of basic biology, translational medicine, biomedicine, and drug development.

Acknowledgements

We would like to thank Professor XF Qi (Jinan University, China), Professor Edouard C. Nice (Monash University, Australia), and Professor Mark Baker (Macquarie University, Australia) for providing assistance and guidance in this project. We specially acknowledge Professor Edouard C. Nice for revising this article.

Conflict of interest

None declared.

Fundings

This work was collectively supported by grants from the Guangdong Innovative and Entrepreneurial Research Team Program (2014ZT05S136), National Key Research and Development Plan (2016YFD0500600), Guangdong Provincial Science and Technology Plan Project (2017B020207004), and Fundamental Research Funds for the Central Universities (21618309).

Acronyms and abbreviations

AAV	adeno-associated virus
APC	adenomatous polyposis coli

ASFV	African swine fever virus
CD163	cysteine-rich domain 163
CRISDA	CRISPR/Cas9-triggered nicking endonuclease-mediated strand displacement amplification
CSFV	classical swine fever virus
gRNAs	guided RNAs
HD	Huntington's disease
HDR	homology-directed recombination
ICSI	intracytoplasmic sperm injection
IGF2	insulin-like growth factor 2
LDLR	low-density lipoprotein receptor
MT/hGH	metallothionein-I/human growth hormone
MSTN	myostatin
PAM	protospacer adjacent motif
PERVs	porcine endogenous retroviruses
PFFs	porcine fetal fibroblasts
PRV	pseudorabies virus
PSCs	pluripotent stem cells
PRRSV	porcine reproductive and respiratory syndrome virus
RNP	ribonucleoprotein
SCNT	somatic cell nuclear transfer
SpCas9	*Streptococcus pyogenes* Cas9
SMG	selectable marker gene
SMGT	sperm-mediated gene transfer
SRSRs	short regularly spaced repeats
T7E1	T7 endonuclease 1
UCP1	uncoupling protein 1
ZAL	zwitterionic amino lipid

Author details

Huafeng Lin[1,2*†], Qiudi Deng[1†], Lili Li[2] and Lei Shi[2]

1 Department of Biotechnology, College of Life Science and Technology, Jinan University, Guangzhou, Guangdong, PR China

2 Institute of Food Safety and Nutrition, Jinan University, Guangzhou, PR China

*Address all correspondence to: 88983088@qq.com

† These authors contributed equally to this work and should be considered co-first authors

References

[1] Krishnasamy V, Otte J, Silbergeld E. Antimicrobial use in Chinese swine and broiler poultry production. Antimicrobial Resistance and Infection Control. 2015;**4**(1):17. DOI: 10.1186/s13756-015-0050-y

[2] USDA. Livestock and Poultry: World Markets and Trade: U.S. Department of Agriculture [Internet]. 2018. Available from: http://www.fas.usda.gov/data/livestock-and-poultry-world-markets-and-trade

[3] Alexandratos N, Jelle B. World agriculture towards 2030/2050: The 2012 revision. Vol. 12. No. 3. Rome: FAO; 2012. ESA Working paper

[4] Swindle MM, Makin A, Herron AJ, Clubb FJ, Frazier KS. Swine as models in biomedical research and toxicology testing. Veterinary Pathology. 2012;**49**:344-356. DOI: 10.1177/0300985811402846

[5] Yanjun W, Li Z, Jing L, Qinyang J, Yafen G, Ganqiu L. Comparative analysis on liver transcriptome profiles of different methods to establish type II diabetes mellitus models in Guangxi Bama mini-pig. Gene. 2018;**6**:1-20. DOI: 10.1016/j.gene.2018.06.014

[6] Kobayashi T, Zhang H, Tang WWC, Irie N, Withey S, Klisch D, et al. Principles of early human development and germ cell program from conserved model systems. Nature. 2017;**546**(7658):416-420. DOI: 10.1038/nature22812

[7] Ishino Y, Shinagawa H, Makino K, Amemura M, Nakata A. Nucleotide sequence of the IAP gene, responsible for alkaline phosphatase isozyme conversion in Escherichia coli, and identification of the gene product. Journal of Bacteriology. 1987;**169**(12):5429-5433. PMID: 3316184

[8] Horvath P, Barrangou R. CRISPR/Cas, the immune system of bacteria and archaea. Science. 2010;**327**:167-170. DOI: 10.1126/science.1179555

[9] Mali P, Esvelt KM, Church GM. Cas9 as a versatile tool for engineering biology. Nature Methods. 2013;**10**(10):957-963. DOI: 10.1038/nmeth.2649

[10] Mojica FJM, Diez-Villasenor C, Soria E, Juez G. Biological significance of a family of regularly spaced repeats in the genomes of archaea Bacteria and Mitochondria. Molecular Microbiology. 2000;**36**(1):244-246. PMID:10760181

[11] Singh A, Chakraborty D, Maiti S. CRISPR/Cas9: A historical and chemical biology perspective of targeted genome engineering. Chemical Society Reviews. 2016;**45**(24):6666. DOI: 10.1039/c6cs00197a

[12] Jansen R, van Embden JDA, Gaastra W, Schouls LM. Identification of genes that are associated with DNA repeats in prokaryotes. Molecular Microbiology. 2002;**43**(6):1565-1575. PMID: 11952905

[13] Nishimasu H, Ran FA, Hsu PD, Konermann S, Shehata SI, Dohmae N, et al. Crystal structure of Cas9 in complex with guide RNA and target DNA. Cell. 2014;**156**(5):935-949. DOI: 10.1016/j.cell.2014.02.001

[14] Hsu PD, Lander ES, Zhang F. Development and applications of CRISPR-Cas9 for genome engineering. Cell. 2014;**157**(6):1262-1278. DOI: 10.1016/j.cell. 2014.05.010

[15] Jiang F, Doudna JA. CRISPR-Cas9 structures and mechanisms. Annual Review of Biophysics. 2017;**46**(1):505-529. DOI: 10.1146/annurev-biophys-062215-010822

[16] Wang HX, Li M, Lee CM, Chakraborty S, Kim HW, Bao G, et al. CRISPR/Cas9-based genome editing for disease modeling and therapy: Challenges and opportunities for nonviral delivery. Chemical Reviews. 2017;**117**(15):9874. DOI: 10.1021/acs.chemrev.6b00799

[17] Sternberg SH, Doudna JA. Expanding the biologist's toolkit with CRISPR/Cas9. Molecular Cell. 2015;**58**(4):568-574. DOI: 10.1016/j.molcel.2015.02.032

[18] Hammer RE, Pursel VG, Rexroad C Jr, Wall RJ, Bolt DJ, Ebert KM, et al. Production of transgenic rabbits. Nature. 1985;**315**(6021):680-683. PMID: 3892305

[19] Whyte JJ, Zhao J, Wells KD, Samuel MS, Whitworth KM, Walters EM, et al. Gene targeting with zinc finger nucleases to produce cloned eGFP knockout pigs. Molecular Reproduction and Development. 2011;**78**:2. DOI: 10.1002/mrd.21271

[20] Carlson DF, Tan W, Lillico SG, Stverakova D, Proudfoot C, Christian M, et al. Efficient TALEN-mediated gene knockout in livestock. Proceedings of the National Academy of Sciences of the United States of America. 2012;**109**(43):17382-17387. DOI: 10.1073/pnas.1211446109

[21] Cong L, Ran FA, Cox D, Lin S, Barretto R, Habib N, et al. Multiplex genome engineering using CRISPR/Cas systems. Science. 2013;**339**:819-823. DOI: 10.1126/science.1231143

[22] Hai T, Teng F, Guo R, Li W, Zhou Q. One-step generation of knockout pigs by zygote injection of CRISPR/Cas system. Cell Research. 2014;**24**(3):372. DOI: 10.1038/cr.2014.11

[23] Whitworth KM, Lee K, Benne JA, Beaton BP, Spate LD, Murphy SL, et al. Use of the CRISPR/Cas9 system to produce genetically engineered pigs from in vitro-derived oocytes and embryos. Biology of Reproduction. 2014;**91**(3):78. DOI: 10.1095/biolreprod.114.121723

[24] Josefsberg JO, Buckland B. Vaccine process technology. Biotechnology and Bioengineering. 2012;**109**:1443-1460. DOI: 10.1002/bit.24493

[25] Wiedenheft B, Sternberg SH, Doudna JA. RNA-guided genetic silencing systems in bacteria and archaea. Nature. 2012;**482**(7385):331-338. DOI: 10.1038/naturc10886

[26] Liang X, Sun L, Yu T, Pan Y, Wang D, Hu X, et al. A CRISPR/Cas9 and Cre/lox system-based express vaccine development strategy against re-emerging pseudorabies virus. Scientific Reports. 2016;**6**:19176. DOI: 10.1038/srep19176

[27] Whitworth KM, Rowland RR, Ewen CL, Trible BR, Kerrigan MA, Cinoozuna AG, et al. Gene-edited pigs are protected from porcine reproductive and respiratory syndrome virus. Nature Biotechnology. 2015;**34**(1):20. DOI: 10.1038/nbt.3434

[28] Xie Z, Pang D, Yuan H, et al. Genetically modified pigs are protected from classical swine fever virus. PLoS Pathogens. 2018;**14**(12):e1007193. DOI: 10.1101/361477

[29] HüBner A, Petersen B, Keil GM, Niemann H, Mettenleiter TC, Fuchs W. Efficient inhibition of African swine fever virus replication by CRISPR/Cas9 targeting of the viral p30 gene (cp204l). Scientific Reports. 2018;**8**(1):1449. DOI: 10.1038/s41598-018-19626-1

[30] Ruan J, Jie X, Chen-Tsai RY, Li K. Genome editing in livestock: Are we ready for a revolution in animal breeding industry? Transgenic Research. 2017;**26**(6):1-12. DOI: 10.1007/s11248-017-0049-7

[31] Wells KD, Prather RS. Genome-editing technologies to improve research, reproduction, and production in pigs. Molecular Reproduction & Development. 2017;**84**(9):1012-1017. DOI: 10.1002/mrd.22812

[32] Whitworth KM, Prather RS. Gene editing as applied to prevention of reproductive porcine reproductive and respiratory syndrome. Molecular Reproduction & Development. 2017;**84**(9):926-933. DOI: 10.1002/mrd.22811

[33] Tao L, Yang M, Wang X, Zhang Z, Wu Z, Tian J, et al. Efficient biallelic mutation in porcine parthenotes using a CRISPR-Cas9 system. Biochemical and Biophysical Research Communications. 2016;**476**(4):225-229. DOI: 10.1016/j.bbrc.2016.05.100

[34] Park KE, Kaucher AV, Powell A, Waqas MS, Sandmaier SE, Oatley MJ, et al. Generation of germline ablated male pigs by CRISPR/Cas9 editing of the NANOS2 gene. Scientific Reports. 2017;7:40176. DOI: 10.1038/srep40176

[35] Klymiuk N, Aigner B, Brem G, et al. Genetic modification of pigs as organ donors for xenotransplantation. Molecular Reproduction & Development. 2010;**77**(3):209-221. DOI: 10.1002/mrd.21127

[36] Hryhorowicz M, Zeyland J, Słomski R, Lipiński D. Genetically modified pigs as organ donors for xenotransplantation. Molecular Biotechnology. 2017;**59**(9):435-444. DOI: 10.1007/s12033-017-0024-9

[37] Ekser B, Ezzelarab M, Hara H, Windt DJVD, Wijkstrom M, Bottino R, et al. Clinical xenotransplantation: The next medical revolution? Lancet. 2012;**379**(9816):672-683. DOI: 10.1016/S0140-6736(11)61091-X

[38] Sato M, Miyoshi K, Nagao Y, Nishi Y, Ohtsuka M, Nakamura S, et al. The combinational use of CRISPR/Cas9-based gene editing and targeted toxin technology enables efficient biallelic knockout of the α-1,3-galactosyltransferase gene in porcine embryonic fibroblasts. Xenotransplantation. 2014;**21**(3):291-300. DOI: 10.1111/xen.12089

[39] Petersen B, Frenzel A, Lucas-Hahn A, Herrmann D, Hassel P, Klein S, et al. Efficient production of biallelic GGTA1 knockout pigs by cytoplasmic microinjection of CRISPR/Cas9 into zygotes. Xenotransplantation. 2016;**23**(5):338-346. DOI: 10.1111/xen.12258

[40] Reyes LM, Estrada JL, Wang ZY, Blosser RJ, Smith RF, Sidner RA, et al. Creating class I MHC-null pigs using guide RNA and the Cas9 endonuclease. Journal of Immunology. 2015;**193**(11):5751-5757. DOI: 10.4049/jimmunol.1402059

[41] Yang L, Güell M, Niu D, George H, Lesha E, Grishin D, et al. Genome-wide inactivation of porcine endogenous retroviruses (PERVs). Science. 2015;**350**(6264):1101-1104. DOI: 10.1126/science.aad1191

[42] Niu D, Wei HJ, Lin L, George H, Wang T, Lee IH, et al. Inactivation of porcine endogenous retrovirus in pigs using CRISPR/Cas9. Science. 2017;**357**(6357):1303. DOI: 10.1126/science.aan4187

[43] Meurens F, Summerfield A, Nauwynck H, Saif L, Gerdts V. The pig: A model for human infectious diseases. Trends in Microbiology. 2012;**20**(1):50-57. DOI: 10.1016/j.tim.2011.11.002

[44] Merrifield CA, Lewis M, Claus SP, Beckonert OP, Dumas ME, Duncker S, et al. A metabolic system-wide characterisation of the pig: A model for human physiology. Molecular BioSystems. 2011;**7**(9):2577. DOI: 10.1039/c1mb05023k

[45] Flisikowska T, Kind A, Schnieke A. Pigs as models of human cancers. Theriogenology. 2016;**86**(1):433-437. DOI: 10.1016/j.theriogenology.2016.04.058

[46] Holm IE, Alstrup AK, Luo Y. Genetically modified pig models for neurodegenerative disorders. Journal of Pathology. 2016;**238**(2):267-287. DOI: 10.1002/path.4654

[47] Zhang Q, Widmer G, Tzipori S. A pig model of the human gastrointestinal tract. Gut Microbes. 2013;**4**(3):193-200. DOI: 10.4161/gmic.23867

[48] Tan W, Carlson DF, Lancto CA, Garbe JR, Webster DA, Hackett PB, et al. From the cover: Efficient nonmeiotic allele introgression in livestock using custom endonucleases. PNAS. 2013;**110**(41):16526-16531

[49] Peng J, Wang Y, Jiang J, Zhou X, Song L, Wang L, et al. Production of human albumin in pigs through CRISPR/Cas9-mediated knockin of human cDNA into swine albumin locus in the zygotes. Scientific Reports. 2015;**5**:16705. DOI: 10.1038/srep16705

[50] Feng W, Dai Y, Mou L, Cooper DK, Shi D, Cai Z. The potential of the combination of CRISPR/Cas9 and pluripotent stem cells to provide human organs from chimaeric pigs. International Journal of Molecular Sciences. 2015;**16**(3):6545-6556. DOI: 10.3390/ijms16036545

[51] Wang X, Cao C, Huang J, Yao J, Hai T, Zheng Q, et al. One-step generation of triple gene-targeted pigs using CRISPR/Cas9 system. Scientific Reports. 2016;**6**:20620. DOI: 10.1038/srep20620

[52] Kang JT, Ryu J, Cho B, Lee EJ, Yun YJ, Ahn S, et al. Generation of RUNX3 knockout pigs using CRISPR/Cas9-mediated gene targeting. Reproduction in Domestic Animals. 2016;**51**(6):970-978. DOI: 10.1111/rda.12775

[53] Zhang W, Wang G, Wang Y, Jin Y, Zhao L, Xiong Q, et al. Generation of complement protein C3 deficient pigs by CRISPR/Cas9-mediated gene targeting. Scientific Reports. 2017;**7**(1):5009. DOI: 10.1038/s41598-017-05400-2

[54] Yan S, Tu Z, Liu Z, Fan N, Yang H, Yang S, et al. A huntingtin knockin pig model recapitulates features of selective neurodegeneration in Huntington's disease. Cell. 2018;**173**(4):989-1002. DOI: 10.1016/j.ccll.2018.03.005

[55] Cho B, Kim SJ, Lee EJ, Ahn SM, Lee JS, Ji DY, et al. Generation of insulin-deficient piglets by disrupting INS gene using CRISPR/Cas9 system. Transgenic Research. 2018;**27**(3):1-12. DOI: 10.1007/s11248-018-0074-1

[56] Arne M, Kirsten J, Mortensen H. Influence of dietary fat on carcass fat quality in pigs. A review. Acta Agriculturae Scandinavica. 1992;**42**(4):220-225

[57] Tomic Z, Stojanac N, Cincovic M, Stevancevic O, Urosevic M, Novakov N, et al. Comparison of the content of lean meat in pigs on farm and slaughter line. Biotechnology in Animal Husbandry. 2018;**34**(1):41-48. DOI: 10.2298/BAH1801041T

[58] Bi Y, Hua Z, Liu X, Hua W, Ren H, Xiao H, et al. Isozygous and selectable marker-free MSTN knockout cloned pigs generated by the combined use of CRISPR/Cas9 and Cre/Loxp. Scientific Reports. 2016;**6**:31729. DOI: 10.1038/srep31729

[59] Zheng Q, Lin J, Huang J, Zhang H, Zhang R, Zhang X, et al. Reconstitution of ucp1 using CRISPR/Cas9 in the white adipose tissue of pigs decreases fat deposition and improves thermogenic capacity. Proceedings of the National Academy of Sciences of the United

States of America. 2017;**114**(45):E9474. DOI: 10.1073/pnas.1707853114

[60] Xiang G, Ren J, Hai T, Fu R, Yu D, Wang J, et al. Editing porcine IGF2 regulatory element improved meat production in Chinese Bama pigs. Cellular and Molecular Life Sciences. 2018;**75**:1-10. DOI: 10.1007/s00018-018-2917-6

[61] Zhou W, Hu L, Ying L, Zhao Z, Chu PK, Yu XF. A CRISPR–Cas9-triggered strand displacement amplification method for ultrasensitive DNA detection. Nature Communications. 2018;**5012, 9**:1-11. DOI: 10.1038/s41467-018-07324-5

[62] Su YH, Lin TY, Huang CL, Tu CF, Chuang CK. Construction of a CRISPR/Cas9 system for pig genome targeting. Animal Biotechnology. 2015;**26**(4):279-288. DOI: 10.1080/10495398.2015.1027774

[63] Ruan J, Li H, Xu K, Wu T, Wei J, Zhou R, et al. Highly efficient CRISPR/Cas9-mediated transgene knockin at the H11 locus in pigs. Scientific Reports. 2015;**5**:14253. DOI: 10.1038/srep14253

[64] Zhou X, Xin J, Fan N, Zou Q, Huang J, Ouyang Z, et al. Generation of CRISPR/Cas9-mediated gene-targeted pigs via somatic cell nuclear transfer. Cellular and Molecular Life Sciences. 2015;**72**(6):1175-1184. DOI: 10.1007/s00018-014-1744-7

[65] Yang Y, Wang K, Wu H, Jin Q, Ruan D, Ouyang Z, et al. Genetically humanized pigs exclusively expressing human insulin are generated through custom endonuclease-mediated seamless engineering. Journal of Molecular Cell Biology. 2016;**8**(2):174-177. DOI: 10.1093/jmcb/mjw008

[66] Wang K, Jin Q, Ruan D, Yang Y, Liu Q, Wu H, et al. Cre-dependent Cas9-expressing pigs enable efficient in vivo genome editing. Genome Research. 2017;**27**(12):2061. DOI: 10.1101/gr.222521.117

[67] Whitworth KM, Cecil R, Benne JA, Redel BK, Spate LD, Samuel MS, et al. Zygote injection of RNA encoding Cre recombinase results in efficient removal of loxp flanked neomycin cassettes in pigs. Transgenic Research. 2018;**27**(1):1-12. DOI: 10.1007/s11248-018-0064-3

[68] Chen F, Wang Y, Yuan Y, Zhang W, Ren Z, Jin Y, et al. Generation of B cell-deficient pigs by highly efficient CRISPR/Cas9-mediated gene targeting. Journal of Genetics and Genomics. 2015;**42**(8):437-444. DOI: 10.1016/j.jgg.2015.05.002

[69] Li P, Estrada JL, Burlak C, Montgomery J, Butler JR, Santos RM, et al. Efficient generation of genetically distinct pigs in a single pregnancy using multiplexed single-guide RNA and carbohydrate selection. Xenotransplantation. 2015;**22**(1):20-31. DOI: 10.1111/xen.12131

[70] Wang X, Zhou J, Cao C, Huang J, Hai T, Wang Y, et al. Efficient CRISPR/Cas9-mediated biallelic gene disruption and site-specific knockin after rapid selection of highly active sgRNAs in pigs. Scientific Reports. 2015;**5**:13348. DOI: 10.1038/srep13348

[71] Chuang CK, Chen CH, Huang CL, Su YH, Peng SH, Lin TY, et al. Generation of GGTA 1 mutant pigs by direct pronuclear microinjection of CRISPR/cas9 plasmid vectors. Animal Biotechnology. 2017;**28**(3):174-181. DOI: 10.1080/10495398.2016.1246453

[72] Whitworth KM, Benne JA, Spate LD, Murphy SL, Samuel MS, Murphy CN, et al. Zygote injection of CRISPR/Cas9 RNA successfully modifies the target gene without delaying blastocyst development or altering the sex ratio in pigs. Transgenic Research. 2017;**26**(1):97-107. DOI: 10.1007/s11248-016-9989-6

[73] Yu HH, Zhao H, Qing YB, Pan WR, Jia BY, Zhao HY, et al. Porcine zygote injection with Cas9/sgRNA results in DMD-modified pig with muscle dystrophy. International Journal of Molecular Sciences. 2016;**17**(10):1668. DOI: 10.3390/ijms17101668

[74] Gao H, Zhao C, Xiang X, Li Y, Zhao Y, Li Z, et al. Production of α-1,3-galactosyltransferase and cytidine monophosphate-N-acetylneuraminic acid hydroxylase gene double-deficient pigs by CRISPR/Cas9 and handmade cloning. Journal of Reproduction and Development. 2017;**63**(1):17-26. DOI: 10.1262/jrd.2016-079

[75] Lei H, Hua Z, Xiao H, Ying C, Xu K, Qian G, et al. CRISPR/Cas9-mediated APOE−/− and LDLR−/− double gene knockout in pigs elevates serum LDL-C and TC levels. Oncotarget. 2017;**8**(23):37751. DOI: 10.18632/oncotarget.17154

[76] Li Z, Yang HY, Wang Y, Zhang ML, Liu XR, Xiong Q, et al. Generation of tryptophan hydroxylase 2 gene knockout pigs by CRISPR/Cas9-mediated gene targeting. The Journal of Biomedical Research. 2017;**12**(5): 445-452. DOI: 10.7555/JBR.31.20170026

[77] Wu J, Vilarino M, Suzuki K, Okamura D, Bogliotti YS, Park I, et al. CRISPR-Cas9 mediated one-step disabling of pancreatogenesis in pigs. Scientific Reports. 2017;**7**(1):10487. DOI: 10.1038/s41598-017-08596-5

[78] Borca MV, Holinka LG, Berggren KA, Gladue DP. CRISPR-Cas9, a tool to efficiently increase the development of recombinant African swine fever viruses. Scientific Reports. 2018;**8**(1):3154. DOI: 10.1038/s41598-018-21575-8

[79] Santos RMND, Reyes LM, Estrada JL, Wang ZY, Tector M, Tector AJ. CRISPR/Cas and recombinase-based human-to-pig orthotopic gene exchange for xenotransplantation. Journal of Surgical Research. 2018;**229**:28-40. DOI: 10.1016/j.jss.2018.03.051

[80] Sato M, Kosuke M, Koriyama M, et al. Timing of CRISPR/Cas9-related mRNA microinjection after activation as an important factor affecting genome editing efficiency in porcine oocytes. Theriogenology. 2018;**108**:29-38. DOI: 10.1016/j.theriogenology.2017.11.030

[81] Yang H, Zhang J, Zhang X, Shi J, Pan Y, Zhou R, et al. CD163 knockout pigs are fully resistant to highly pathogenic porcine reproductive and respiratory syndrome virus. Antiviral Research. 2018;**151**:63-70. DOI: 10.1016/j.antiviral.2018.01.004

[82] Song M. The CRISPR/Cas9 system: Their delivery, in vivo and ex vivo applications and clinical development by startups. Biotechnology Progress. 2017;**33**(4):1035-1045. DOI: 10.1002/btpr.2484

[83] Choi JG, Dang Y, Abraham S, Ma H, Zhang J, Guo H, et al. Lentivirus pre-packed with Cas9 protein for safer gene editing. Gene Therapy. 2016;**23**(7): 627-633. DOI: 10.1038/gt.2016.27

[84] Deng Q, Chen Z, Shi L, Lin H. Developmental progress of CRISPR/Cas9 and its therapeutic applications for HIV-1 infection. Reviews in Medical Virology. 2018;**28**(5):1-7. DOI: 10.1002/rmv.1998

[85] Gori JL, Hsu PD, Maeder ML, Shen S, Welstead GG, Bumcrot D. Delivery and specificity of CRISPR-Cas9 genome editing technologies for human gene therapy. Human Gene Therapy. 2015;**26**(7):443. DOI: 10.1089/hum.2015.074

[86] Yin H, Kanasty RL, Eltoukhy AA, Vegas AJ, Dorkin JR, Anderson DG. Non-viral vectors for gene-based therapy. Nature Reviews Genetics. 2014;**15**(8):541-555. DOI: 10.1038/nrg3763

[87] Li L, He ZY, Wei XW, Gao GP, Wei YQ. Challenges in CRISPR/Cas9 delivery: Potential roles of nonviral vectors. Human Gene Therapy. 2015;**26**(7):452. DOI: 10.1089/hum.2015.069

[88] Roth TL, Puigsaus C, Yu R, Shifrut E, Carnevale J, Hiatt J, et al. Reprogramming human T cell function and specificity with non-viral genome targeting. Nature. 2018;**559**:405-409. DOI: 10.1038/s41586-018-0326-5

[89] Lino CA, Harper JC, Carney JP, Timlin JA. Delivering CRISPR: A review of the challenges and approaches. Drug Delivery. 2018;**25**(1):1234-1257. DOI: 10.1080/10717544.2018.1474964

[90] Ryu J, Prather RS, Lee K. Use of gene-editing technology to introduce targeted modifications in pigs. Journal of Animal Science and Biotechnology. 2018;**9**(1):5. DOI: 10.1186/s40104-017-0228-7

[91] Kabadi AM, Ousterout DG, Hilton IB, Gersbach CA. Multiplex CRISPR/Cas9-based genome engineering from a single lentiviral vector. Nucleic Acids Research. 2014;**42**(19):e147-e147. DOI: 10.1093/nar/gku749

[92] Zhang Z, Wan T, Chen Y, Sun H, Cao T, et al. Cationic polymer-mediated CRISPR/Cas9 plasmid delivery for genome editing. Macromolecular Rapid Communications. 2019;**40**(5):1800068. DOI: 10.1002/marc.201800068

[93] Ehrke-Schulz E, Schiwon M, Leitner T, Dávid S, Bergmann T, Liu J, et al. CRISPR/Cas9 delivery with one single adenoviral vector devoid of all viral genes. Scientific Reports. 2017;7(1):17113. DOI: 10.1038/s41598-017-17180-w

[94] Liu C, Zhang L, Liu H, Cheng K. Delivery strategies of the CRISPR-Cas9 gene-editing system for therapeutic applications. Journal of Controlled Release. 2017;**266**:17-26. DOI: 10.1016/j.jconrel.2017.09.012

[95] He ZY, Men K, Qin Z, Yang Y, Xu T, Wei YQ. Non-viral and viral delivery systems for CRISPR-Cas9 technology in the biomedical field. Science China Life Sciences. 2017;**60**(5):458-467. DOI: 10.1007/s11427-017-9033-0

[96] Yin H, Xue W, Chen S, Bogorad RL, Benedetti E, Grompe M, et al. Corrigendum: Genome editing with Cas9 in adult mice corrects a disease mutation and phenotype. Nature Biotechnology. 2014;**32**(9):952-952. DOI: 10.1038/nbt.2884

[97] Xue W, Chen S, Yin H, et al. CRISPR-mediated direct mutation of cancer genes in the mouse liver. Nature. 2014;**514**:380-384. DOI: 10.1038/nature13589

[98] Lee K, Conboy M, Park HM, Jiang F, Kim HJ, Dewitt MA, et al. Nanoparticle delivery of Cas9 ribonucleoprotein and donor DNA in vivo induces homology-directed DNA repair. Nature Biomedical Engineering. 2017;**1**(11):889. DOI: 10.1038/s41551-017-0137-2

[99] Sun W, Ji W, Hall JM, et al. Self-assembled DNA nanoclews for the efficient delivery of CRISPR-Cas9 for genome editing. Angewandte Chemie International Edition. 2015;**54**(41):12029-12033. DOI: 10.1002/anie.201506030

[100] Watanabe M, Nagashima H. Genome editing of pig. Methods in Molecular Biology. 2017;**1630**:121

[101] Polejaeva IA, Chen SH, Vaught TD, Page RL, Mullins J, Ball S, et al. Cloned pigs produced by nuclear transfer from adult somatic cells. Nature. 2000;**407**:86-90. DOI: 10.1038/35024082

[102] Ma H, Young M, Yang Y. Somatic-cell nuclear transfer (SCNT). Stem Cells. 2014;**5**(4):12-21

[103] Wang L, Wu J, Fang W, JCI B, et al. Regenerative medicine: Targeted genome editing in vivo. Cell Research. 2015;**25**:271-272. DOI: 10.1038/cr.2015.11

[104] Hao Y, Song CQ, Dorkin JR, Zhu LJ, Li Y, Wu Q, et al. Therapeutic genome editing by combined viral and non-viral delivery of CRISPR system components in vivo. Nature Biotechnology. 2016;**34**(3):328-333. DOI: 10.1038/nbt.3471

[105] Kang XJ, Caparas CIN, Soh BS, Fan Y. Addressing challenges in the clinical applications associated with CRISPR/Cas9 technology and ethical questions to prevent its misuse. Protein and Cell. 2017;**8**(11):1-5. DOI: 10.1007/s13238-017-0477-4

[106] Kumar M, Keller B, Makalou N, Sutton RE. Systematic determination of the packaging limit of lentiviral vectors. Human Gene Therapy. 2001;**12**(15):1893. DOI: 10.1089/104303401753153947

[107] Rossi A, Salvetti A. Integration of AAV vectors and insertional mutagenesis. Medecine/Sciences. 2016;**32**(2):167-174. DOI: 10.1051/medsci/20163202010

[108] Zincarelli C, Soltys S, Rengo G, Rabinowitz JE. Analysis of AAV serotypes 1–9 mediated gene expression and tropism in mice after systemic injection. Molecular Therapy. 2018;**16**:1073-1080. DOI: 10.1038/mt.2008.76

[109] Chew WL, Tabebordbar M, Cheng JKW, et al. A multifunctional AAV–CRISPR–Cas9 and its host response. Nature Methods. 2016;**13**(10):868. DOI: 10.1038/nmeth.3993

[110] Mout R, Ray M, Lee YW, Scaletti F, Rotello VM. In vivo delivery of CRISPR/Cas9 for therapeutic gene editing: Progress and challenges. Bioconjugate Chemistry. 2017;**28**(4):880-884. DOI: 10.1021/acs.bioconjchem.7b00057

[111] Wang Y, Du Y, Shen B, Zhou X, Li J, Liu Y, et al. Efficient generation of gene-modified pigs via injection of zygote with Cas9/sgRNA. Scientific Reports. 2015;**5**:8256. DOI: 10.1038/srep08256

[112] Zhang XH, Tee LY, Wang XG, Huang QS, Yang SH. Off-target effects in CRISPR/Cas9 mediated genome engineering. Molecular Therapy Nucleic Acids. 2015;**4**(11):e264. DOI: 10.1038/mtna.2015.37

[113] Zischewski J, Fischer R, Bortesi L. Detection of on-target and off-target mutations generated by CRISPR/Cas9 and other sequence-specific nucleases. Biotechnology Advances. 2017;**35**(1):95. DOI: 10.1016/j.biotechadv.2016.12.003

[114] Ihry RJ, Worringer KA, Salick MR, Frias E, Ho D, Theriault K, et al. P53 inhibits CRISPR–Cas9 engineering in human pluripotent stem cells. Nature Medicine. 2018;**24**:939-946. DOI: 10.1038/s41591-018-0050-6

[115] Haapaniemi E, Botla S, Persson J, Schmierer B, Taipale J. CRISPR/Cas9 genome editing induces a p53-mediated DNA damage response. Nature Medicine. 2018;**24**:927-930. DOI: 10.1038/s41591-018-0049-z

Chapter 3

Possible Production of Genome-Edited Animals Using Gene-Engineered Sperm

Masahiro Sato and Shingo Nakamura

Abstract

CRISPR/Cas9 is widely used for genome editing in a variety of organisms, including mammals, fishes, and plants. In mammals, zygotes are considered an appropriate target for gene delivery of CRISPR/Cas9 components [Cas9 endonuclease and a single-guide (sgRNA)] via microinjection or *in vitro* electroporation. However, these approaches require *ex vivo* handling of zygotes, which is necessary for egg transfer to recipient females to allow the treated zygotes to develop full-term. These procedures are often laborious, time-consuming, and use numerous mice. In our previous experiments, the plasmid DNA encapsulated by liposomal reagent introduced into the internal portion of a testis can be transferred to the mature sperm present in the epididymal ducts, and is finally transferred to oocytes via fertilization. Although it was not integrated into their genome, this approach would be useful for creating genome-edited animals, since CRISPR/Cas9 can be performed by transient interaction of Cas9 and sgRNA, whereby chromosomal integration of the CRISPR components is not a prerequisite. Here, we will review past achievements concerning in vivo transfection of immature/mature sperm and present experimental proposals for possible genome editing via gene-engineered sperm based on recent findings.

Keywords: sperm, CRISPR/Cas9, guide RNA, testis-mediated gene transfer, *in vivo* transfection, genome editing, vas deferens, epididymis, artificial insemination, intratesticular injection

1. Introduction

Transgenesis is a method to induce genetic change in an organism by delivering exogenous DNA (also called transgenes) to early embryos (i.e., zygotes), and is now considered an important technique to examine gene function *in vivo* and for creating animal models of human disease [1, 2]. In 1980, Gordon et al. [3] first demonstrated that microinjection of purified DNA fragments into the pronuclei of zygotes led to the production of mice carrying the transgenes, which are generally referred to as transgenic (Tg) or genetically modified (GM) mice. When the injected transgenes are successfully integrated into the host chromosomes of the zygotes, they are transmitted to the next generation through mating with normal mice in a Mendelian ratio, and gene expression derived from the integrated transgenes will occur in the Tg offspring depending on the property of the promoter used. For the production of Tg animals through zygote microinjection, several steps are required for the "*ex vivo* handling of embryos," including: collection of zygotes, DNA microinjection using an expensive micromanipulator, temporal incubation of the injected zygotes, and egg transfer (ET) to the oviducts of the pseudo-pregnant females to allow full-term development of the injected eggs [4, 5]. Furthermore, all of this requires highly specialized and skilled personnel for the preparation of pseudo-pregnant females and vasectomized males, which is time-consuming and tedious, and requires a large number of mice.

Since 1980, several methods for bypassing microinjection-based transgenesis have been provided, which include infection of zygotes with viral vectors like a retrovirus [6, 7], embryonic stem (ES) cell-based gene transfer [8–10], transgenesis via somatic cell nuclear transfer [11–13], and intracytoplasmic sperm injection (ICSI) using sperm associated with the transgene (TransICSI) [14, 15]. All of these methods deal with zygotes and require *ex vivo* handling of embryos, although a micromanipulator system is not used in almost the cases.

Genome-editing via Oviductal Nucleic Acids Delivery (GONAD) is a recently developed method for creating GM mice and rats without *ex vivo* handling of embryos [16–21]. It can be simply performed by injecting a solution containing nucleic acids into the oviductal lumen of pregnant females at zygote to two-cell stages and subsequent *in vivo* electroporation (EP) to enhance DNA uptake by early embryos *in situ*. In this case, there is no need for the large number of mice that is normally required for the traditional microinjection-based transgenesis: only four to five pregnant females are required for modifying an endogenous gene [18]. Thus, creation of GM animals is simplified with the development of GONAD, but an expensive apparatus electroporator is still required for the technique.

In 1989, Lavitrano et al. [22] reported the simplest, convenient, and cost-effective method to create GM animals, which was called sperm-mediated gene transfer (SMGT), where isolated sperm were incubated in the presence of naked plasmid DNA for a short period and these DNA-associated sperm were subjected to *in vitro* fertilization (IVF) with normal oocytes. The resulting progeny are later judged as those carrying the exogenous DNA in their genome. Since the report, there has been controversy over its reproducibility among researchers [23–25]. However, several recent improvements were made on this SMGT system by several researchers who employed reagents capable of enhancing gene delivery towards isolated sperm [26–28]. For example, Shen et al. [29] incubated mouse sperm in a solution containing 3% dimethyl sulfoxide (DMSO) and plasmid DNA for 10–15 min at 4°C prior to IVF. Embryos (42%; 25/60) obtained from this experiment showed bright enhanced green fluorescent protein (EGFP)-derived fluorescence. Furthermore, Kim et al. [30] reported that nanoparticles, such as magnetic nanoparticles, can be a vehicle for delivering exogenous DNA to sperm from various animals such as boar. They incubated boar sperm in the presence of 0.5% (v/v) of magnetic nanoparticles (MNPs) and plasmid DNA coding for green fluorescent protein (GFP) on the magnetic field for 90 min, and the magnetofected sperm were subjected to IVF with normal oocytes. As a result, they obtained fertilized eggs expressing GFP. Unfortunately, for further development of IVF-derived embryos, it still required ET towards recipient females, which is laborious and requires specialized skill. Notably, it is possible to perform artificial insemination (AI) using *in vitro*-transfected sperm, which can be simply done by injecting those sperm into the uterine horn or lumen of the oviducts of recipient females showing oocyte ovulation. This method, called "SMGT-based AI" (SMGT-AI), has already been performed by several laboratories and will be discussed in more detail in the last part of this paper.

Testis-mediated gene transfer (TMGT) is the *in vivo* version of SMGT, in which sperm is transfected *in vivo*. This technology was first developed by Sato et al. [31], who performed intratesticular injection of calcium phosphate-precipitated plasmid DNA using a glass micropipette in mice. The injected exogenous DNA is transferred to epididymal sperm or spermatogenic cells within a seminiferous tubule (ST) of the testis, and those transfected sperm will transmit it to an oocyte through fertilization (**Figure 1**). They could detect the injected DNA in isolates of sperm from the epididymis and from the uteri of females mated with the injected males, but the DNA could not be detected in embryos [31]. In contrast with SMGT, TMGT does not require *ex vivo* handling of embryos such as collection of oocytes, IVF and ET. In this context, TMGT appears to be more convenient and simpler than SMGT for the purpose of GM animal production. Since the report of Sato et al. [31], several *in vivo* gene delivery approaches targeted to male reproductive systems have been reported: gene delivery to spermatogenic cells by intratubular injection of STs (ST-mediated gene transfer, STGT) (**Figure 2a**), to epididymal sperm present in the epididymal ducts (epididymis-mediated gene transfer, EpiGT) (**Figure 2b**), and to sperm present in the vas deferens (vas deferens-mediated gene transfer, VDGT) (**Figure 2c**).

Based on this background, the previous terminology TMGT appears to be now recognized as "direct *in vivo* gene delivery approach towards male reproductive system." In this context, it may be better to re-name TMGT as "intratesticular injection-based gene transfer" (IIGT), which involves direct injection of genetic materials into the interstitial space of a testis. Thus, IIGT, STGT, EpiGT and VDGT can be considered as TMGT-related experiments. In **Table 1**, a summary of previous studies on TMGT-related experiments is listed. Furthermore, there are several excellent papers reviewing the SMGT/TMGT-related studies [28, 90–93], which provide a helpful survey of this field.

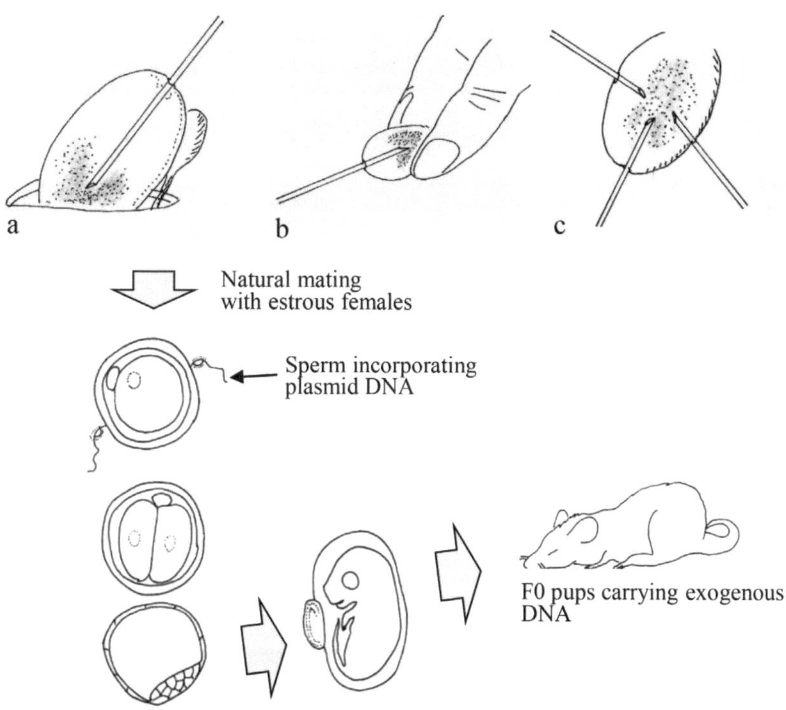

Figure 1.
IIGT in mice. To perform IIGT, at least three different ways to inject a DNA-containing solution into the testis have been employed. The first way (shown in a) is to perform IIGT towards a testis (that is exposed outside after surgery) under anesthesia [31, 32]. The second way (shown in b) is to perform IIGT through insertion of a needle via scrotum under anesthesia [33]. The third way (shown in c) is to insert a needle at three times to different sites [34]. In these latter two cases, no surgery is required. Three to five days after IIGT, the IIGT-treated males are subjected to mating with normal estrous females. The in vivo transfected sperm may fertilize ovulated oocytes, leading to creation of offspring carrying the introduced exogenous DNA.

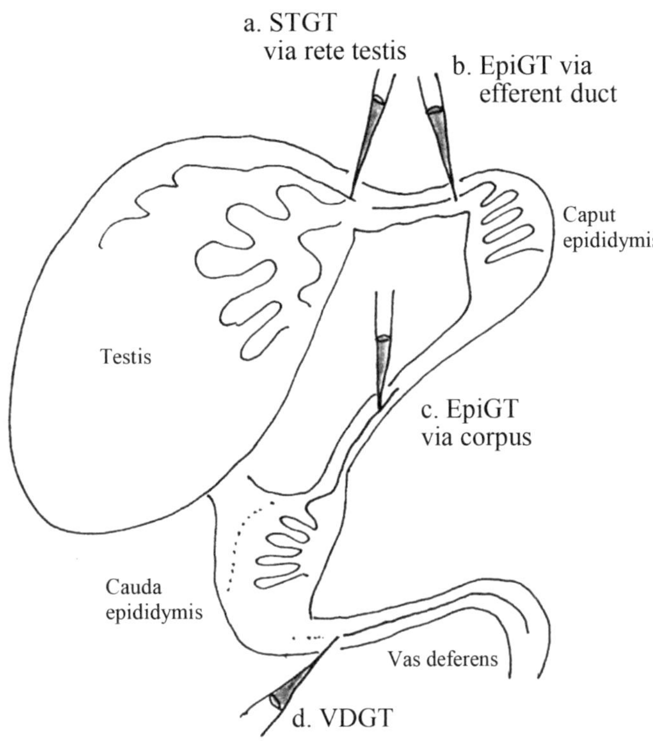

Figure 2.
There are several routes for introducing exogenous DNA into the male reproductive system. The routes for DNA injection are as follows: (a) STGT via rete testis; (b) EpiGT by inserting a glass pipette into the proximal region of caput epididymis; (c) EpiGT by inserting a glass pipette into the proximal region of cauda epididymis; and (d) VDGT by inserting a glass pipette into the proximal region of vas deferens.

Method	Species	DNA/transfection method	Outcome (note)	References
IIGT	Mice	Plasmid/calcium phosphate	The exogenous DNA was detectable in the sperm isolated from caput and cauda epididymides as early as 6 h after IIGT and in the ejaculated sperm from the female uteri, but not in 1-cell eggs	[31]
IIGT	Mice	Plasmid/liposome/IIGT 3 times at 4-day intervals	Eighty percent of blastocysts expressed lacZ from the exogenous DNA, suggesting successful transmission of the exogenous DNA to F0 offspring	[34]
IIGT	Rats	Adenovirus	Leydig cells expressed the transgene	[35]
IIGT	Mice	Plasmid/EP	Some spermatogenic-like cells expressed the transgene	[36]
IIGT	Mice	Plasmid/liposome/2–5 days after IIGT, the males were mated to females	Transmitted the foreign DNA to F0 offspring at frequencies of 4.3–92.3%; the copy number of the exogenous DNA was estimated to be less than 1 copy per diploid cell; no transgene expression in mid-gestational F0 fetuses	[32]

Method	Species	DNA/transfection method	Outcome (note)	References
IIGT	Mice	Plasmid/liposome/2 days after IIGT, the males were mated to females	Transmitted the foreign DNA to F0 offspring at frequencies of 50.0–84.6%; expression of lacZ in most (71.9%) blastocysts, but no expression of foreign DNA in the mid-gestational F0 fetuses; transmission of the exogenous DNA from F0 to F1 generation at frequencies from 16.1–23.1%, suggesting that the introduced DNA was chimeric in these F0 mouse testes	[33]
IIGT	Mice/rats	Plasmid/liposome/3–4 days after IIGT, the males were mated to females	Transmitted the foreign DNA to F0 offspring at frequencies of 18% in rats and 20% in mice; transgene expression in F0 offspring; transmission of the exogenous DNA up to F4 generation	[37]
IIGT	Mice/rats	Plasmid/liposome/4 days after IIGT, the males were mated to females	Detection of exogenous DNA in the head and tail of epididymal sperm; also, in the ejaculated sperm isolated from the female uteri; failure to detect the exogenous DNA in the DNase-treated sperm, suggesting no integration of the transgene in sperm DNA	[38]
IIGT	Mice	Plasmid/liposome/2 days after IIGT, the males were mated to females	Although seven commercially available transfection reagents were tested for possible improvement of IIGT to increase copy number of transgenes integrated and transgene expression, drastic improvement failed; transgene expression indeed occurred, but the degree of its expression diminished with development; choice of reagents used appears not to be so critical for IIGT	[39]
IIGT	Rats	Plasmid/liposome/4 days after IIGT, the males were mated to females	Detection of foreign DNA (encapsulated by DMRIE-C and SuperFect among eight liposomes tested) in sperm in the cauda epididymis isolated 1, 4, and 14 days after IIGT; more than 80% of morulae expressed EGFP; the ratio of animals carrying the foreign DNA decreased as they developed, suggesting high incidence of mosaicism	[40]
IIGT	Mice	Plasmid (lacZ/retroviral integrase gene)/EP	One month after IIGT, some spermatocyte-like cells in STs expressed the lacZ gene; co-transfection with integrase gene resulted in prolonged expression of lacZ, suggesting the usefulness of integrase gene co-transfection for stable transformation of spermatogenic cells *in vivo*	[41]

Method	Species	DNA/transfection method	Outcome (note)	References
IIGT	Mice	TB or Hoechst 33342/ plasmid/EP	TB was rapidly transported to the epididymal portion after IIGT; TB reached the corpus and cauda epididymis within 2–4 days after injection; sperm isolated from epididymal portion had the exogenous DNA even after DNase I treatment, suggesting incorporation of the DNA inside the sperm	[42]
IIGT	Mice	Adenovirus	Presence of the transgenes in sperm from 7 to 16 days after inoculation; transgenes are detected in the sperm heads in oocytes after IVF; the transgene product was mainly present in the interstitial tissue of a testis; it was also present in the STs and collected sperm; the transgene product was located in the head and the mid-piece of sperm	[43]
IIGT	Fishes (silver sea bream)	Plasmid/liposome	IIGT was performed 48 h before spawning. After mating these IIGT-treated males to females, between 59 and 76% of the hatched fry were found to be Tg; the efficiency of gene transfer was improved more than 80% by injecting multiple doses of the transgenes; Southern blot analysis showed that the transgene was integrated into the host genome	[44]
IIGT	Mice	Plasmid/EP	To study regulatory elements of genes specifically active in spermatocytes, IIGT-EP was performed; in the EP-based IIGT-treated testes, only small fraction of cells expressed the transgenes; this method can be useful for preliminary screening of constructs aimed to study in Tg mice	[45]
IIGT	Mice	Adenovirus/IIGT at 3 sites per testis	The transgene expression was found in Leydig cells, but no expression was noted in germ cells	[46]
IIGT	Mice	Plasmid/liposome/repeated injections (singly, 3 or 6 times 3 days apart)	Repeated injections of the exogenous DNA led to a high rate of gene transfer, but failed to introduce high numbers of copies (more than 1 copy per diploid cell); expression of transgene-derived mRNA was observed, although its strength appeared still to be very low	[47]
IIGT	Mice	Plasmid/liposome/3 times 3 days apart/7–21 days after IIGT, the males were mated to females	Detection of the presence of at least two types of the exogenous DNA, intact and deleted form of plasmid in F0 offspring, suggesting degradation of the exogenous DNA during the process of IIGT	[48]

Method	Species	DNA/transfection method	Outcome (note)	References
IIGT	Mice	Plasmid/EP	LacZ activity was detected in spermatogenic cells up to 4 weeks after IIGT	[49]
IIGT	Mice	Adenovirus/EP	EP might be effective for transfecting germ cells or somatic cells	[50]
IIGT	Mice	Plasmid/PEI	Transferred and expressed in germ cells (especially in primary spermatocytes); transfection into Sertoli cells was not observed; protein showed dynamic shifts in spermatogenic cells at different stages during spermatogenesis	[51]
IIGT	Mice/ rabbits	Plasmid/DMSO	F0 offspring (mice) expressed EGFP with an efficiency of 28.6%; also 56.3% of rabbits born were identified to be Tg	[29]
IIGT	Shellfishes (Japanese abalone)	Naked plasmid (linearized)	The gene-transfer efficiency of G_0 in larvae (9 h after fertilization), juveniles (3 weeks after fertilization), and 1-year-old adults was 90%, 92.5%, and 60%, respectively; genomic Southern blot analysis showed that the transgene was integrated in the genome of the Tg abalone	[52]
IIGT	Mice	Linearized plasmid/liposome (DOTAP)/IIGT at multi-sites/ after few weeks, the males were mated	41% of F0 offspring exhibited the presence of the transgenes when PCR and Southern blot hybridization were employed; 37% of F1 offspring obtained after mating of F0 offspring with wild-type mice were Tg	[53]
IIGT	Mice	Linearized plasmid/EP	Successful gene delivery to undifferentiated spermatogonia within the STs; about 94% of females after mating with the IIGT-treated males successfully sired Tg pups	[54]
IIGT	Chickens	Plasmid/cationic polymer	The percentages of gene expression reached the summit and became stable from day 70 to 160, being 12.7%, 12.8%, 15.9% and 19.1%, respectively; Southern blot showed that the transgene was inserted in their genomic DNAs	[55]
IIGT	Chickens	Plasmid for EGFP-lacZ dual reporter expression/liposome (Lipofectamine 2000)	Ten days post-IIGT, fluorescent sperms were not observed on semen slides; however, sperms positive for lacZ were detected; specific amplicons of EGFP and lacZ detectable in four of the six sequentially collected semen samples; staining with monoclonal antibodies demonstrated positive staining for subsets of testicle cells	[56]

Method	Species	DNA/transfection method	Outcome (note)	References
IIGT	Mice	Plasmid/DMSO, DMA or liposome (Lipofectin)/1 day after IIGT, each male was mated	The presence of transgene in the progeny (80% for PCR positive when repeated injection was done; 50% for RT-PCR positive) in the case of liposome was used; 55.5% for PCR positive, but 22.3% for RT-PCR positive in the case of DMSO was used; RT-PCR analysis of PCR positive animals showed EGFP expression in blood cells; repeated (4 times) injections of DNA complexes can affect spermatogenesis	[57]
IIGT	Mice	Plasmid/liposome (Lipofectamine 2000)/6 weeks after IIGT, each male was mated	38.46% of F0 positive for transgenes in the case of PCR; 30.77% by Southern blotting; 36.36% of F1 were positive for the transgene; expression of EGFP is recognized	[58]
IIGT	Mice	Plasmid/liposome (ExGen500)/at different angles into the testes of 7-day-old males	Transgene efficiencies were 11.76% (2/17), 14.29% (3/21), and 11.11% (2/18), respectively; semi-quantitative RT-PCR analysis further showed that the introduced GFP gene was expressed in 3/9 integration mice; GFP expression was observed in sperm from the F0 fetuses and F1 pups	[59]
IIGT	Mice	Linearized plasmid/EP	Electroporated testis expressed EGFP even 80 days after IIGT; EGFP expressing germ cells were discernible in the STs; after mating with the EP-based IIGT-treated males with normal females, the resultant Tg pups showed tissue-specific expression of transgene	[60]
IIGT	Mice	Plasmid/liposome (PEI)	Twenty days after IIGT, the transgene-derived fluorescence was detected in the testis and sperm; foreign DNA was successfully expressed in the treated mice: 4.0% for G0 and 30.23% for F1	[61]
IIGT	Mice	Plasmid/liposome (DOTAP)	The Tg positive rate in mouse F1 offspring was 39.69%; gene transmission beyond F2 generation; the transgene was expressed in the ovaries	[62]
IIGT (*in vitro*)	goats	Plasmid/EP	Cultivation (organ culture) of STs isolated from the IIGT-EP-treated testis led to expression of GFP 24 h after EP; green fluorescence was observed at best 23 days after EP-based IIGT	[63]
IIGT	Rats	GFP-expressing plasmid/EP	Possible integration of transgene into the genome of the spermatogonial cells; a transgenic disease model displaying alpha thalassemia was successfully generated with EP-based IIGT	[64]

Method	Species	DNA/transfection method	Outcome (note)	References
IIGT	Mice	Linearized Plasmid/hypotonic Tris-HCl solution	Successful internalization of the transgene in spermatogonia within STs; such IIGT-treated males generated Tg progeny by natural mating	[65]
IIGT	Mice	Plasmid/BMPs-PEI	DNA complexed with BMPs-PEI successfully reached the cytoplasm and the nucleus of spermatogenesis cell; the transgene was expressed in the testes of Tg F0 mice; the ratio of Tg F0 offspring was 88%	[66]
IIGT	Goats	Plasmid/EP	Successful transfer of the transgene into STs and testicular cells; chromosomal integration of the transgene and its expression in sperm; natural mating of a pre-founder buck produced a Tg baby goat	[67]
STGT	Mice/pigs	Plasmid/liposome (obtained from Gibco)	In mice, 8.0–14.8% of STs expressed the introduced LacZ gene, and 7–13% of epididymal sperm had the foreign DNA; in pigs, foreign DNA was also incorporated into male germ cells, and 15.3–25.1% of the STs containing germ cells expressed the LacZ gene	[68]
STGT	Rats	Adenovirus	Expression of the transgene in Sertoli cells and persisted for at least 10 days	[35]
STGT	Mice	Plasmid/EP	Specific lacZ expression only in haploid spermatid cells; spermatogenic differentiating cells maintained the transfected lacZ expression after more than 2 months of transfection, suggesting that spermatogenic stem cells and/or spermatogonia could also incorporate foreign DNA	[69]
STGT	Mice	Plasmid/EP	Transient expression of GFP in the innermost region of the testis uniformly, but confined to spermatogenic cells and Sertoli cells within the STs; GFP was detected in the spermatogenic cells even 2 months after EP; no Tg offspring were obtained	[70]
STGT	Mice	Plasmid/EP	After EP-based STGT, fluorescent sperm were collected from the STGT-treated STs; these fluorescent sperm were found to have the ability to produce Tg offspring, when ICSI was performed	[71]
STGT	Mice	adeno-, adeno-associated-, retro-, and lentiviral vectors	Transduction with either adeno- or lentiviral vectors led to reporter gene expression for more than 2 months after STGT; lentiviral vectors used to express the c-kit ligand in Sl/Sl(d) Sertoli cells restored spermatogenesis; lentiviral vectors failed to infect spermatogenic cells	[72]

Method	Species	DNA/transfection method	Outcome (note)	References
STGT	Mice	Plasmid/EP	By electrotransformation of a complete cDNA in Sertoli cells, defective spermatogenesis was rescued in infertile Sl(17H)/Sl(17H) mutant mice	[73]
STGT	Mice	Plasmid/liposome (noncommercial cationic lipids)	As early as 48–96 h post-injection, lacZ expression was observed within both immature and differentiated germ cells; by 40 days post-injection, it was restricted to the most immature germ cells; after mating with females, the transgene was transmitted to the offspring, but remained episomal	[74]
STGT	Mice	Adenovirus	Strong expression in Sertoli cells after STGT, but no expression in germ cells	[46]
STGT	Mice	Retrovirus	Transduction of spermatogonial stem cells with an average efficiency of 2.8%; the transgene was transmitted stably and expressed in the next generation	[75]
STGT	Mice	Plasmid/EP	STGT was performed to examine testis-specific gene promoter activity; successful *in vivo* transient transfection to living mouse testis was achieved	[76]
STGT	Mice	Plasmid/EP	LacZ activity was detected in spermatogenic cells up to 8 weeks after EP-based SMGT	[49]
STGT	Hamsters	Plasmid/EP	Sixty days following gene transfer, expression of the transgene can be detected in epididymal sperm	[77]
STGT	Mice	Plasmid/EP	The transgene products were found on the head and mid-piece regions of mature epididymal sperm	[78]
STGT	Mice	Plasmid/EP	A fluorescent reporter protein expressed in male germ cells	[79]
STGT	Mice	Plasmid RNAi targeting EGFP/EP	Sertoli cells were the main transfected cells	[80]
STGT	Mice	Plasmid/EP	STGT is useful for testing the tissue-specific promoter activity included in the construct *in vivo*	[81]
STGT	Mice	Adenovirus	Sertoli cell-specific expression of GFP	[82]
STGT	Mice	Lentivirus	All male pre-founder mice produced Tg pups with an overall success rate of over 60%	[83]
STGT	Mice	Lentivirus	14.3% of the lentivirus-injected mice successfully produced Tg pups; eight Tg founders were obtained from the total 336 pups; the Tg efficiency was around 2.4%	[84]
EpiGT	Rats	Plasmid/EP	After 72 h, the initial segments had intense fluorescence in the cytoplasm of the epithelial cells	[85]

Method	Species	DNA/transfection method	Outcome (note)	References
EpiGT	Mice	Plasmid/lipid (FuGENE 6)	Transfection was observed in 39.70% of epithelial cells after 2 days and in 31.77% after 7 days; the presence of the transgene in the DNA isolated from the treated epididymides (by PCR); GFP gene expression appeared in large areas of the cauda epididymis even after 2 weeks post-EpiGT	[86]
VDGT	Mice/rats	Plasmid	Uptake of exogenous DNA occurred in 60–70% of the spermatozoa after *in vitro* or *in vivo* treatments; positive signal was detected in the sperm nucleus and was not affected by DNase treatment	[87]
VDGT	Mice	Mixture of linearized and circular plasmids	From 53 newborns, four were found positive by PCR for the GFP gene; some tissues showed expression for GFP	[88]
VDGT	Mice	Plasmid/liposome (Lipofectamine)	Maximum of 6.8% in the epithelial cells of the vas (for lacZ staining); 13.3% after employing the GFP gene construction; expression of the GFP gene appeared from 1 week up to 3 months following injection	[89]

[1]*TMGT can be defined as a method for in vivo gene delivery towards male reproductive systems (testis, epididymis, and vas deferens) and includes intratesticular injection-based gene transfer (IIGT), seminiferous tubule-mediated gene transfer (STGT), epididymis-mediated gene transfer (EpiGT), and vas deferens-mediated gene transfer (VDGT).*
Abbreviations: BMPs, bacterial magnetic particles; DMSO, dimethyl sulfoxide; DOTAP, N-[1-(2,3-Dioleoyloxy) propyl]-N,N,N-trimethylammonium methyl sulfate; DMA, N,N-dimethylacetamide; EP, electroporation; GFP, green fluorescent protein; IVF, in vitro fertilization; PEI, polyethylenimine; STs, seminiferous tubules; Tg, transgenic; TB, trypan blue.

Table 1.
Summary of testis-mediated gene transfer (TMGT)[1]-related studies.

In the following sections, the TMGT-related experiments will be mentioned in more detail.

2. Historical background of TMGT-related experiments

2.1 IIGT-related experiments

Between 1994 and 2006, over 20 reports on IIGT-related experiments were reported using various animal models such as mice, rats, hamsters, rabbits, boar, goats, chicks, fishes, and shellfishes [29, 31–41, 43–53, 68]. The DNA used were mainly plasmid DNA that had been mixed with calcium phosphate, liposomes/lipids, polyethylenimine (PEI), or DMSO, all of which were intended to facilitate uptake of DNA by sperm or spermatogenic cells [29, 31–34, 37–40, 44, 47, 48, 51, 68]. The method to use *in vivo* EP towards the entire testis after IITG with naked plasmid DNA was also employed [36, 41, 45, 49]. Furthermore, adenoviral vectors were introduced by IIGT [35, 43, 46, 50].

Through these works, the following information became available:

i. **Transgene expression in a testis after IIGT:** IIGT using an adenoviral vector resulted in preferential transgene expression in Leydig cells [46]. Mogas et al. [43] reported that transgene-derived protein is mainly present in the interstitial tissue of a testis, and in STs 7–16 days after inoculation. Li et al. [51] demonstrated that plasmid DNA mixed with PEI can be transferred within STs after IIGT and expressed in primary spermatocytes, but not Sertoli cells.

ii. **Detection of transgenes and expressed products on the epididymal or ejaculated sperm:** According to Yonezawa et al. [40], foreign DNA encapsulated by DMRIE-C and SuperFect can be detected by PCR in the cauda epididymis-derived sperm isolated 1, 4, and 14 days after IIGT. The exogenous DNA was also detectable in the ejaculated sperm collected from the uterine horn of the females in the morning after mating with the IIGT-treated males [31, 38].

iii. **Transgene expression in the F0 offspring obtained after mating with the IIGT-treated males:** PCR analysis revealed that detection of the transgenes in the mid-gestational fetuses was found at frequencies ranging about 50–85% [39]. However, the copy number of the transgenes in those fetal DNA are estimated to be <1 copy per diploid cell [32]. PCR/slot blot analyses revealed that 41% of F0 offspring had the transgenes [53]. Ogawa et al. [34] reported that 80% of blastocysts exhibited the transgene-derived lacZ gene coding for β-galactosidase, one of the key enzymes consisting of lactose operon. Sato et al. [39] reported that lacZ expression was evident in most (72%) of the blastocysts, but neither expression of the LacZ gene nor its mRNA was found in the mid-gestational fetuses. More than 80% of morulae expressed EGFP, but the ratio of animals carrying the foreign DNA decreased as they developed, and only some of the progeny were foreign DNA-positive with high incidence of mosaicism [40].

iv. **Transgene transmission to the next generation:** Gene transmission to F1 offspring was at frequencies ranging about 16–23%, but when F2 offspring was obtained from mating normal female with F1 male offspring, about 94% of F2 offspring had the transgenes, suggesting that the introduced DNA was chimeric in these F0 mouse testes [38]. On the contrary, He et al. [53] demonstrated that the transgene transmission rate from F0 to F1 generation was 37%, suggesting that the transgene transmission rate was similar to the Mendelian law of inheritance.

In 2007 and onward, attempts to improve IIGT systems were made by several laboratories to enhance the gene delivery efficiency [54–67]. In the following sections, we will describe several examples [(v) to (x)] about the improvement of IIGT, *in vitro* assessment for gene expression after IIGT or possible mechanism underlying IIGT.

v. **IIGT at a young stage:** In mammalian testis, spermatogenesis occurs in the STs of a testis (**Figure 3d**). In the ST, there are spermatogenic cells called spermatogonia (spermatogonial cells) that can be further matured into spermatocytes and spermatids. Spermatogonia are largely divided into two types, type A and type B cells. The former undergoes active mitosis and divide to produce type B cells. The type B cells divide to give rise to spermatocytes and spermatids, which move towards the lumen of the ST as they mature. According to Hui-ming et al. [59], type A spermatogonia first appear between 3 and 7 days postnatally in mice and are the only immortalized diploid cells. They considered that if these type A spermatogonia are stably transfected with the exogenous DNA, the transfected cells would be able to produce mature Tg sperm leading to production of Tg mice through natural fertilization. Based on this hypothesis, they performed IIGT using GFP-expressing plasmid DNA encapsulated by the ExGen500 transfection reagent on 7-day old male ICR mice. When these treated mice reached different stages of sexual maturity (6, 12, and 24 weeks of age), they were mated with normal females. The resulting pups were identified as Tg, with efficiencies of 11–14%. They observed GFP expression in sperm cells isolated from F0 and F1 pups. They referred to this technology as "type A spermatogonia-mediated gene transfer" (TASMGT).

vi. **EP-based IIGT:** Majumdar's group developed a method for generating Tg mice by directly injecting the desired gene into the testis followed by *in vivo* EP [54]. In this method, one of the testis was surgically exposed for DNA injection (**Figure 1a**) and the other contra-lateral testis was removed. An improved version of this EP-based IIGT was provided by Usmani et al. [60], who introduced the transgenes to both testes of mice directly from the outside (**Figure 3a**), prior to *in vivo* EP. They employed a two-step EP in which four 60 V electric pulses (50 ms each with an inter-pulse interval of 1 s) in one direction (forward direction) (**Figure 3b**) and four more pulses after changing the sides of the electrodes (reverse direction) (**Figure 3c**). The EP-based IIGT-treated testis expressed EGFP from the introduced transgenes even at 80 days of age. Furthermore, fluorescent germ cells were discernible in the STs of those mice (**Figure 3d**). F1 offspring that were generated after mating the IIGT-EP-treated males with normal females showed tissue-specific expression of transgenes. This improved procedure is based on non-surgical gene delivery using a two-step EP, which appears to be a user-friendly technique for a person who is less experienced in performing surgery.

vii. ***In vitro* EP-based IIGT:** It is difficult to apply IIGT in the testis of larger animals such as goats, because the size of the testis is much bigger than that of smaller animals such as mice and rats. Raina et al. [63] hypothesized that IIGT may be possible when *in vitro* gene delivery is performed towards the testis dissected from goats. They slowly injected GFP-expressing plasmid DNA into the interstitial space at eight different sites of the isolated testis using a 1-mL syringe (**Figure 4a**). Then, the testis was subjected to *in vitro* EP using a pair of tweezer-type electrodes (**Figure 4b**). After that, ST was partially dissociated and placed under *in vitro* cultivation for checking GFP expression at regular intervals (**Figure 4c, d**). A strong green fluorescence signal was observed 24 h after EP and its expression was continuously observed for as long as 23 days post-EP. The authors mention that the results of this study cannot be applied straightforwardly for *in vivo* studies, but the *in vitro* transfection of ST using EP will provide valuable baseline information, prior to IIGT *in vivo*.

viii. **IIGT using a simple hypotonic solution:** Majumdar's group have developed a method to generate Tg mice by directly injecting the desired gene in the testis followed by *in vivo* EP, as mentioned above [54, 60]. This technique is less complicated for small animal like mice but appears to not be feasible for transgenesis in large animals, because these animals have larger testes and greater scrotal thickness, to which it is difficult to standardize voltage parameters. To overcome this difficulty, they developed an alternative technique for making Tg mice by hypotonic shocking male germ cells for gene delivery. According to Usmani et al. [65], treatment with hypotonic Tris-HCl solution reduced osmolarity and led to hypotonic-swelling of germ cells. The hypotonic-swelling eventually killed the cells with increased hypotonicity, but led to the uptake of surrounding molecules

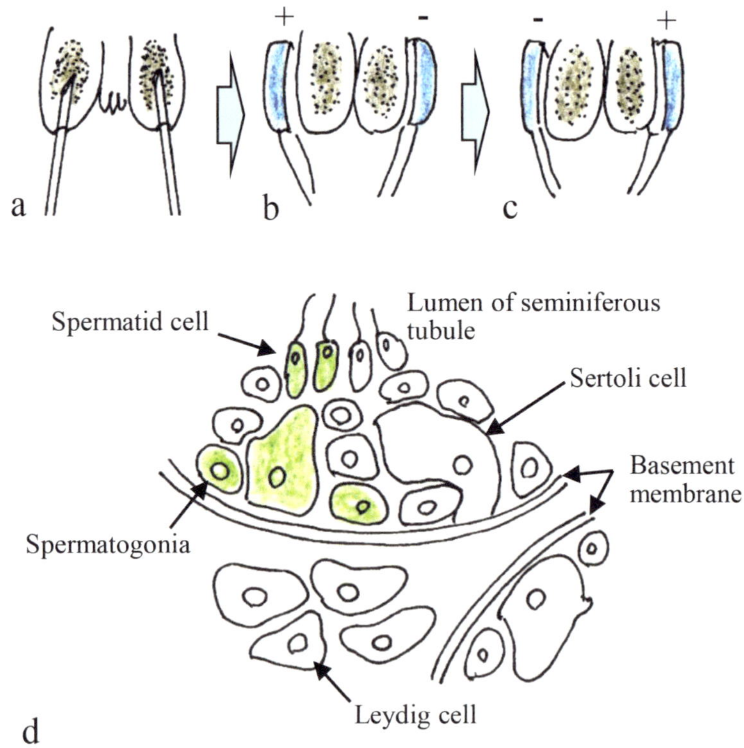

Figure 3.
EP-based IIGT in mice. a-c. Schematic illustration for EP-based IIGT. After IIGT towards both testes (a), they are held by a pair of tweezer-type electrodes and then subjected to the first in vivo EP (b). The second EP was next performed by changing the direction of electric pulse (c). (d) Structure of a ST. The colored spermatogenic cells and Sertoli cells indicate cells successfully transfected by the exogenous DNA that have been instilled within a lumen of ST.

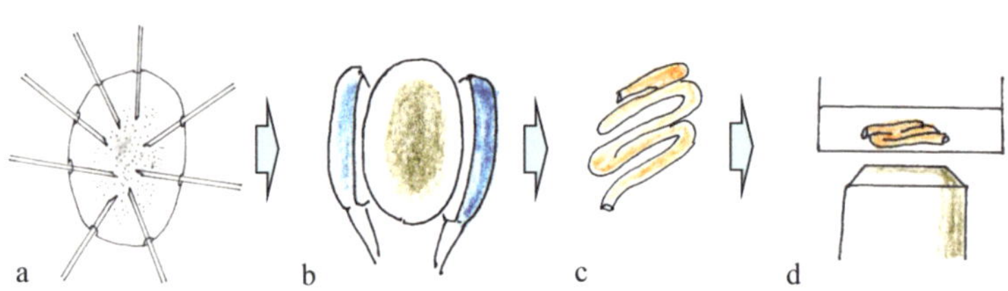

Figure 4.
In vitro EP-based IIGT in goats. The isolated goat testis is subjected to IIGT with a total of eight repeated injections from different directions (a). Then, the entire testis is hold by a pair of electrodes prior to EP (b). After that, the EP-treated STs are partially dissected and subjected to in vitro cultivation (c). By this, the transgene expression on the spermatogenic cells of STs can be monitored continuously (d).

such as nucleosides inside the cell. The authors hypothesized that a hypotonic Tris-HCl solution at a certain hypotonic concentration might allow the germ cells to internalize the surrounding solutes like DNA *in vivo* without being killed and the sperm produced from transfected germ cells may carry a desired DNA fragment (transgene) to generate Tg animals. Usmani et al. [65] suspended the linearized plasmid DNA (transgenes) in hypotonic Tris-HCl solution (pH 7.0) and simply performed IIGT to internalize the injected transgenes in the genome of spermatogonia residing at basal compartment of tubules. As a result, such males successfully generated Tg progeny by natural mating. This technique is easy and simple and does not require expensive apparatuses like electroporators. Usmani et al. [65] proposed that such a procedure enables researchers to generate their own Tg animals, instead of outsourcing, and would drastically minimize the time required for studies on functional genomics.

ix. **IIGT using nanoparticles:** It has previously been reported that nanoparticles such as magnetic nanoparticles, mesoporous silica nanoparticles, and halloysite clay nanoparticle can be used as a vehicle for delivering exogenous DNA to sperm of various animals, such as boar and bovine [30, 94–96]. However, these early reports are confined to *in vitro* events. Wang et al. [97] applied this technology to IIGT using bacterial magnetic particles (BMPs)/PEI complex-conjugated foreign DNAs (BMP-PEI-DNA complex). According to Wang et al. [97], BMPs help to reduce the toxicity of the PEI, an efficient gene transfer agent, and assist gene delivery *in vivo*. After performing IIGT in mice, the testis was returned to the original position, and a neodymium-iron-boron magnet with an intensity of 600 milliteslas (mT) was placed onto the surface of the abdomen to facilitate gene delivery towards the spermatogenic cells. The authors report that this procedure is not harmful to the functioning of the testis. They reported that the clusters of BMP-PEI-DNA complex successfully reached the cytoplasm and the nucleus of spermatogenic cell and expressed in the testes of F0 mice. The resulting F0 mice could transmit the introduced transgene to the offspring with efficiencies of 88%.

x. **Possible mechanism for IIGT-mediated gene delivery to sperm:** When intratesticular injection of a DNA-containing solution into the interstitial space of a testis is performed, the fate of the injected solution is largely divided into two routes. This was first assessed by Sato et al. [42] who employed trypan blue (TB) as dye to visualize the transferring solution. One route is when a solution is transferred to the epididymal ducts, and the other route is when a solution is transferred to the lumen of the STs (**Figure 5**). After the intratesticular injection of 30 μL TB, the dye was rapidly transferred via rete testis to the proximal segment of caput epididymis [42]. One day after the injection, the dye was observed in the middle segment of caput epididymis. This was also confirmed by a previous observation using PCR analysis, which revealed the presence of the exogenous DNA in the spermatozoa isolated from caput epididymis [31]. Furthermore, the exogenous DNA can be detected in the ejaculated sperm collected from the uterine horn 1 day after mating with females [31]. Thus, it is reasonable to consider that the exogenous DNA injected into the interstitial space of a testis is rapidly transferred to the epididymal ducts and taken up by epididymal sperm *in situ*.

Only a minor portion of the solution injected into the interstitial space of a testis is transferred inside the STs. This may be elicited by mechanical shearing of STs upon insertion of a needle or glass capillary. To increase the transfection efficiency in the spermatogenic cells existing within STs, repeated needle insertions (over at least three times from different sites) have been employed by some research groups [34, 46, 53, 59, 63]. At present, it remains unknown how many STs are indeed transfected by this treatment. Usmani et al. [65] reported that spermatogenic cells, including spermatogonia present within STs, are transfected after IIGT and subsequent *in vivo* EP using fluorescent marker genes.

2.2 STGT-related experiments

ST is a tubular structure packed in a testis, which contains spermatogenic cells, such as spermatogonia, a precursor for mature sperm, and maturing sperm cells

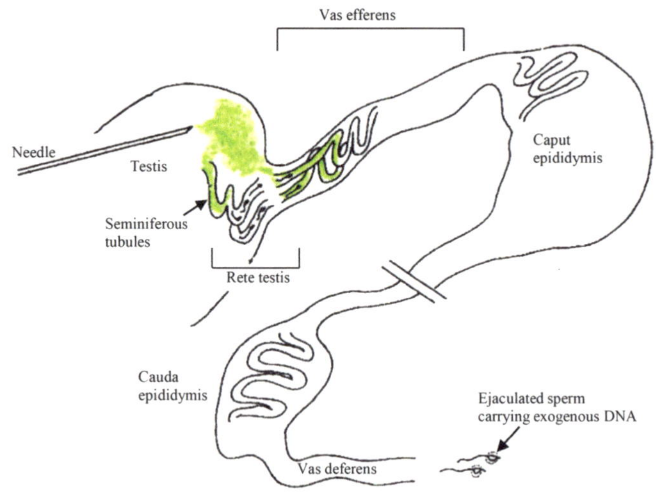

Figure 5.
Possible mechanism of how the exogenous DNA introduced into the interstitial space of a testis is transmitted to epididymal sperm or to spermatogenic cells within a ST.

(spermatocytes and spermatids), and Sertoli cells, which support the proliferation and differentiation of spermatogonia (**Figure 3d**). If the exogenous DNA is introduced within a lumen of the ST, it is possible to transfect those spermatogenic cells, from which transfected spermatozoa are transported via epididymal ducts and finally ejaculated upon mating with estrous females. As a result, the introduced exogenous DNA will be transmitted to oocytes via fertilization with the transfected sperm.

To our knowledge, STGT was first performed in 1997 by two groups: Blanchard and Boekelheide [35], with rats using adenoviral vector, and Kim et al. [68], with mouse and pigs using liposomally encapsulated plasmid DNA. The aim of the former group was to study transgene expression in the adult rat testis *in vivo*. They demonstrated that there was transgene expression in Sertoli cells and principal cells of the epididymis, and expression persisted for at least 10 days. The latter group demonstrated that in mice, 8.0–14.8% of STs expressed the introduced transgene, as evaluated by histochemical staining for the lacZ gene, and 7–13% of epididymal sperm had the exogenous DNA, as evaluated by PCR analysis. In pigs, 15–25% of the STs contained lacZ-positive germ cells. They suggested that STGT can be used as a powerful tool for producing Tg livestock.

In 1998, Yamazaki et al. [69] employed STGT for examining transcriptional regulatory elements of spermatogenic specific genes. After injecting DNA into STs, subsequent *in vivo* EP was used to enhance DNA uptake by spermatogenic cells. Based on these experiments, they suggested that spermatogenic stem cells and/or spermatogonia can incorporate foreign DNA, and that the transgene could be transmitted to the progenitor cells derived from a transfected proliferating germ cell. Later, the same group [70] examined the possibility to create Tg offspring using STGT coupled with *in vivo* EP (EP-based STGT). Although long-lasting transgene expression could be detected in the spermatogenic cells even 2 months after EP, no Tg offspring were obtained after natural mating with normal adult females.

Huang et al. [71] used the EP-based STGT towards an entire mouse testis after intratubular injection of plasmid DNA that coded for fluorescent genes. To trace the fate of transfected spermatogenic cells, they obtained fluorescent sperm by fluorescence activated cell sorting (FACS), and performed ICSI to obtain their offspring. Almost all the individuals produced from fluorescent sperm were Tg. The authors claim that this is the first report of gene transfer into germ cells and subsequent production of Tg offspring.

STGT appears to be the direct approach to transfect spermatogenic cells *in situ*, but most experiments [46, 49, 51, 72–84] have been confined to successful transfection of spermatogenic cells and Sertoli cells for rescuing damaged/inactive Sertoli cells, *in vivo* testing of efficiency of RNA interference (RNAi), or establishment of an *in vivo* assay system to evaluate the promoter activity of the gene of interest. There have been no trials to create Tg offspring through STGT. Only some groups have tried to test the possibility of creating Tg animals by STGT. For example, Celebi et al. [74] performed STGT using circular plasmid carrying the lacZ reporter gene mixed with noncommercial cationic lipids. These injected males were mated with wild-type females and the progeny were analyzed by PCR and Southern blot assay. They demonstrated that the transgenes were transmitted to the offspring, but remained episomal, since it was found in the tail of the young animals and was lost at adulthood. Therefore, the plasmid seemed to be lost during the numerous germ cell divisions. This plasmid stayed in some tissues, such as in the skeletal and cardiac muscles. No integrative forms have yet been found with the use of circular DNA. Kanatsu-Shinohara et al. [75] described a novel approach for producing Tg animals by transducing spermatogonial stem cells *in vivo* using a retroviral vector by STGT. When these injected males were mated with wild-type females, Tg offspring were obtained with an efficiency of 2.8%. The transgene was transmitted stably and expressed in the next generation. The authors, thus, concluded that this technique will be useful as an alternative to the pre-exiting microinjection-based transgenesis, as well as provide a means for analyzing the self-renewal and differentiation processes of spermatogonial stem cells *in vivo*. Sehgal et al. [83] described a technique for the generation of Tg mice by infection of spermatogonial stem cells with recombinant lentiviruses expressing EGFP with a high rate of success. When the infected males were mated to normal females, over 60% of the delivered pups were found to be Tg. Li et al. [84] employed methods similar to those of Kanatsu-Shinohara et al. [75] and Sehgal et al. [83] and reported that the Tg efficiency is around 2.4%, which is similar to the previous report of Kanatsu-Shinohara et al. [75].

2.3 EpiGT-related experiments

Epididymal sperm present on the ducts of caput and cauda epididymides and epididymal epithelial cells can be targeted for transfection by the exogenous DNA. Kirby et al. [85] performed intraluminal injections (2–5 μL) of plasmid DNA into the lumen of an initial segment tubule of caput epididymis (**Figure 2b**), and subsequent *in vivo* EP towards the injected portion to examine the function of epididymal epithelial cells, which are thought to play critical role in sperm maturation during transport through epididymides. They concluded that this procedure is useful for elucidating the activity of promoter elements included in the injected plasmid that may not be identified when traditional *in vitro* methods are used. Esponda and Carballada [86] injected plasmid DNA mixed with the lipid FuGENE6 into the lumen of mouse cauda epididymis (**Figure 2c**). Successful transfection was observed in about 40% of cells after 2 days and in about 32% after 7 days, and then diminished progressively over time. Gene expression continued up to 15 days after gene injection and occupied about 22% of the area of the tubules. They concluded that intraluminal injections of exogenous DNA are effective for the study of epididymal physiology or to change the fertilizing ability of sperm. These studies are not aimed to create Tg animals, but they hold a potential to transfect epididymal sperm as a useful Tg tool.

2.4 VDGT-related experiments

In 1998, the Esponda's group [87] first attempted to examine whether exogenous plasmid DNA introduced into the lumen of the proximal region of the vas deferens could be taken up by mouse and rat sperm (**Figure 2d**). They demonstrated that 60–70% of sperm recovered 6 h after DNA injection had positive signal for successful transfection in their sperm nucleus, which was not affected by DNase treatment. This was also confirmed by PCR and slot blot analyses. They concluded that sperm within the vas deferens had the ability to incorporate exogenous DNA, which can be transferred to their nuclei, and vas deferens secretions do not block these capacities. In 2000, the same group [88] showed that this VDGT is useful for production of Tg mice. They injected plasmid DNA encoding GFP into the lumen of mouse vas deferens. The night after injections, males were mated with normal estrous females, and the offspring were analyzed. About 8% (4/53) of the newborns delivered expressed the GFP gene. They concluded that VDGT is a simple alternative to the pre-existing microinjection-based production of Tg animals and can be used for species in which the microinjection procedure is not feasible. This technology was later found to also be useful for transfection of epithelial cells of the vas deferens using a direct injection of DNA-liposome complexes, which could modify vas fluid contents [89].

3. Historical background of SMGT-based AI

As mentioned previously, AI of transfected sperm with exogenous DNA through SMGT is a highly convenient route for producing Tg animals. To our knowledge, Sperandio et al. [98] was the first to demonstrate its usefulness in domestic animals, such as bovine and swine. They performed AI towards ten sows with boar sperm cells that had been preincubated with plasmid DNA and obtained 82 offspring. Southern blot analysis of the DNA extracted from the animal tails showed that five animals were Tg and contained sequences complementary to the exogenous plasmid DNA that appeared to be rearranged compared to the original plasmid. From this study, it was suggested that SMGT-AI can be successfully adapted for the generation of Tg livestock. Yonezawa et al. [99] tested whether liposome-peptide (derived from human protamine)-DNA complex (LPD), a new reagent known to stabilize transfection in cultured cells, was useful to increase the efficiency of SMGT. They performed AI using rat epididymal sperm that had been incubated in a solution containing GFP expressing plasmid DNA and LPD complex. Expression of GFP was detectable in the morulae isolated from the treated animals. Furthermore, the AI-treated animals produced pups carrying foreign DNA.

This SMGT-AI is applicable to avian species. Yang et al. [100] performed AI using freshly-ejaculated chicken sperm that had been incubated in the presence of plasmid DNA and liposome, and found that about 4% (2/53) newly hatched chicks was identified as Tg. Harel-Markowits et al. [101] employed restriction enzyme-mediated insertion (REMI) to increase the efficacy of the transfection towards the isolated chicken sperm. REMI was used to insert exogenous DNA linearized with a restriction enzyme that cuts the genomic DNA at sites that enable the exogenous DNA to integrate via its matching cohesive ends [102, 103]. Following insemination with sperm transfected with linearized DNA, restriction enzyme, and liposome, they obtained Tg offspring. Furthermore, when chicken sperm are incubated in a solution containing plasmid DNA and DMSO or N,N-dimethylacetamide (DMAc) and subsequently subjected to AI, the resultant newborn chicks have the transgene, with efficiencies of 38% (for the DMSO-treated group) and 19% (for the

DMAc-treated group) [104]. However, Chaparian et al. [105] recently reported that they were unable to create Tg chicks by SMGT-AI.

4. Exosomes as a possible carrier to deliver genetic materials to sperm

Exosomes, membrane-enclosed sub-cellular microvesicles shed from most cell types, are present in a wide variety of body fluids [106]. Recently, it was found that they can mediate various effects on the behavior of recipient cells, since they contain cytokines, growth factors, and membrane proteins [107]. Furthermore, they contain a substantial amount of small and functional RNA molecules, called microRNAs (<100 nucleotides in length) [108], which could potentially control gene expression of various endogenous genes. It has recently been shown that these exosomes are (1) found in human semen [109], (2) involved in sperm maturation process during the transit along the male epididymal tracts [110], (3) accumulated in mature spermatozoa nuclei [111], and (4) delivered to oocytes through fertilization [112].

Notably, there are some reports describing non-Mendelian germline-independent inheritance of phenotypes in the absence of any classically identifiable mutation or predisposing genetic lesion in the genome of individuals who develop the disease [113–115]. For example, Cossetti et al. [116] performed subcutaneous inoculation of EGFP-expressing human melanoma cells into an immunocompromised mouse, from which EGFP RNA was released from the grafted melanoma cells, delivered to the bloodstream, and finally brought to sperm. When epididymal sperm isolated from these tumor-bearing males were examined carefully, the EGFP RNA was found to be tightly associated with the extracellular fraction of these mature sperm. They termed this phenomenon "soma-to-germ line transmission of information," and thought that exosomes may be involved in this phenomenon as the carrier to deliver EGFP RNA. The findings of Cossetti et al. [116] appear to be well correlated with those obtained from the TMGT-related experiments done at earlier stages of IIGT development, which include (1) non-Mendelian transmission of the exogenous DNA in the offspring obtained [33], (2) extreme low copy number of the exogenous DNA (<1 copy per diploid cell) transmitted to these offspring [32], (3) mosaic expression of the exogenous DNA in the offspring (blastocysts) obtained [33, 40], and (4) reduction in the number of offspring carrying the exogenous DNA during development [40]. As mentioned in Section 2.1 (x), parts of a solution introduced into the interstitial space of a testis is transferred to the excurrent ducts of epididymides, and the exogenous DNA may be taken up by the extracellular fraction of epididymal sperm, possibly through exosomes. We detected the presence of exogenous DNA in the DNase I-treated epididymal sperm, which have been isolated from the IIGT-treated males [42]. This may be due to the fact that exosomes can protect its exogenous DNA against DNase I-mediated digestion.

Notably, in their review article, Jiang and Gao [117] demonstrated that exosomes can be used as naturally occurring cell-to-cell transporters or as novel biocarriers for gene and drug delivery. These exosomes are naturally secreted by the cells and pass through additional biological barriers. They are more biocompatible and biodegradable and can avoid immune response which is most likely due to the surface expression of the complement regulatory proteins, such as CD55 and CD59. For these natural characteristics, exosomes are being extensively explored as gene delivery vehicles. For example, in 2011, Alvarez-Erviti et al. [118] first demonstrated that exosomes are useful for delivering short interfering (si)RNA to the mouse brain. They engineered dendritic cells to express lysosome-associated membrane protein 2 (Lamp2) isoform (Lamp2b), an exosomal membrane protein fused to a neuron-specific peptide. Following that, exosomes were isolated from the gene-engineered dendritic cells and loaded with siRNA using electroporation and were administered intravenously to mice. As a result, the targeting peptide was shown to be successfully delivered to the brain. The concomitantly delivered siRNA caused reduced expression of a target protein associated with the pathogenesis of Alzheimer's disease. Furthermore, Lin et al. [119] proposed that exosomes can be a good carrier to introduce various cargoes, including plasmid DNA, into a cell. They prepared a mixture composed of purified exosomes isolated from HEK293FT cell line, pEGFP-C1 plasmid DNA, and Lipofectamine 2000 liposomes *in vitro*. During the incubation at 37°C for 12 h, exomes and liposomes are fused together and the exogenous plasmid DNA becomes incorporated into exosome-liposome hybrid nanoparticles. Transfecting mesenchymal stem cells (MSCs), which cannot be transfected by the liposome alone, with this complex resulted in successful generation of fluorescent cells when evaluated by FACS. Now, an exosome-based transfection kit, possibly based on this principle, is commercially available: Exo-Fect Exosome Transfection Kit (System Biosciences). We confirmed the usefulness of this kit by *in vivo* transfecting oviductal epithelial cells through intraoviductal instillation of a solution prepared using this kit. Some oviductal epithelial cells were found to be fluorescent after transfection with a plasmid expressing GFP (unpublished results). Thus, it may be possible to transfect isolated sperm by incubating plasmid DNA and exosome/liposome hybrid vesicles provided from the Exo-Fect Exosome Transfection Kit, prior to AI as mentioned below.

5. Genome-editing sperm

Gene modification based on recently developed techniques such as zinc-finger nucleases (ZFNs), TAL effector nucleases (TALENs), and clustered regularly interspersed short palindromic repeats/CRISPR-associated protein 9 (CRISPR/Cas9) are now recognized as a revolutionary genetic engineering tool *in vitro* and *in vivo* [120–124]. Three types of endonucleases from ZFNs, TALENs, and CRISPR/Cas9 have been developed to promote precise genome editing at a target gene. All these enzymes have a DNA-binding ability and an ability to elicit double-strand DNA break (DSB) at a target genomic locus. Subsequently, in the absence of a homologous template to repair, nonhomologous end joining (NHEJ) occurs and causes small insertions or deletions (termed "indels"). In the presence of a template donor DNA, site-specific recombination through homology-directed repair (HDR) occurs. Generally, the frequency of NHEJ is thought to be higher than that of HDR in most of the cell types [125]. **Table 2** shows comparison among these three technologies.

ZFNs are the first engineered endonucleases [127] that combine the DNA recognition ability of zinc-finger protein (called zinc-finger motifs) and restriction enzyme *Fok I* to introduce DSB [120–124]. In 2005, Urnov et al. [128] first demonstrated that ZFNs are effective as a genome editing system in the human cells.

TALENs are similar to ZFNs and require a string of TALEN motif (consisting of a series of 33–35 amino acid repeats) to bind to the specific sequence of a target gene and *Fok I* enzyme to introduce DSB [120–124]. TALENs provide more flexibility to the target sequences since ZFNs are known to be more active towards GC-rich region, whereas TALENs can be assembled to the target AT-rich regions [120–124].

Since both ZFNs and TALENs require assembling of an array to build each set, which is a complex and time-consuming process [124], CRISPR/Cas9 has become the favorite because of its easy application. CRISPR/Cas9 requires only two components,

	ZFN	TALEN	CRISPR/Cas9
Working mechanism	DNA/protein interaction	DNA/RNA/protein interaction	DNA/RNA/protein interaction
Core components	TALE and *Fok* I fusion protein	TALE and *Fok* I fusion protein	Cas9 protein and sgRNA
Design	Easy	Easy	Very easy
Construction	Easy	Easy	Very easy
Efficiency	High	High	High
Off-target rate	Low	High	High

[1] *Based on Chen and Gao [126].*

Table 2.
Comparison of ZFN, TALEN, and CRISPR/Cas9-mediated genome editing systems[1].

the Cas9 nuclease and a single-guide RNA (sgRNA), which is a short sequence to guide the Cas9 protein to a target site. More importantly, these events are performed by transient interaction of Cas9 and sgRNA, whereby chromosomal integration of the CRISPR components is not a prerequisite [129]. There is a concern of off-target cleavage activity from the endonuclease from CRISPR/Cas9 because the system requires recognition of only 20 bp target sequence and allows up to 5 bp mismatches for the formation of DSB [124]. Several strategies for minimizing the off-target cleavage have been employed including use of double nickase mutant form of Cas9, which induces a single-strand break instead of DSB [130]; use of Cas9-sgRNA ribonucleoprotein (RNP) complex, whose half-life is shorter than that the time in which plasmid or viral nucleic acid is transcribed [131]; or use of fusions of catalytically inactive Cas9 with *Fok* I nuclease domain (fCas9) to improve the DNA cleavage specificity [132].

In the case of producing GM animals using SMGT or TMGT, it is better for the exogenous DNA (transgenes) to be integrated into the chromosomes of sperm. This event appears to occur more frequently in immature sperm cells present in the ST of a testis than in the mature epididymal sperm because the chromosomal DNA in the latter cells is tightly packed in the head region of a sperm. In this context, STGT is a preferable system to create GM animals because it is targeted to transfection of spermatogenic cells present within the STs. However, it takes about 4 weeks for mature sperm to reach the epididymal portion for fertilization. If a researcher wants to generate GM animals within a short period of time, direct transfection of mature sperm present in epididymides or vas deferens is recommended. In this case, as mentioned above, the introduced exogenous DNA may be associated to the extracellular fraction of a sperm, as episomal DNA. Notably, CRISPR/Cas9-based genome editing does not always require chromosomal integration of its components; it can be performed by transient expression of their components after transfection [129]. In this sense, an attempt to transfect mature sperm would be a useful alternative for GM animal production.

6. Proposal of new experimental systems for simple creation of genome-edited animals using *in vivo* or *in vitro* transfected sperm

In the following section, we propose two experimental plans to create genome-edited animals using VDGT or AI-based systems, all of which are simpler and more convenient than the previously described systems.

6.1 VDGT-based genome editing

As previously described in Section 2.4, VDGT enables transfer of exogenous DNA to oocytes via fertilization by mature sperm transfected within vas deferens [87, 88]. Injecting a solution containing genome editing components (e.g., sgRNA + DNA/mRNA/protein for Cas9) into the lumen of vas deferens of anesthetized males and subsequent mating between the VDGT-treated males and normal estrous females the day (night) after the surgery may result in production of genome-edited offspring.

In **Figure 6a–c**, experiments obtained after TB injection into the lumen of mouse vas deferens is shown (unpublished results). Under anesthesia, cauda epididymis and vas deferens were pulled out and a small slit was made at the proximal region of vas deferens using micro scissors (**Figure 6a**). Then, a glass micropipette containing TB was inserted into the lumen of vas deferens under observation using a dissecting microscope and about 15 μL of the solution is slowly injected (**Figure 6b**). It is easily discernible that the injected TB still remains within the proximal portion of vas deferens immediately after the injection (arrows in **Figure 6c**). However, the injected TB moved to the distal portion of vas deferens the next day (arrow in **Figure 6d**). Thus, to produce genome-edited animals by VDGT, a solution containing CRISPR/Cas9 components (sgRNA + DNA/mRNA/protein for Cas9), gene delivery enhancing reagents (such as DMSO, liposomes, microparticles, etc.) and fluorescent marker expression plasmid DNA has to be prepared first (**Figure 6e**).

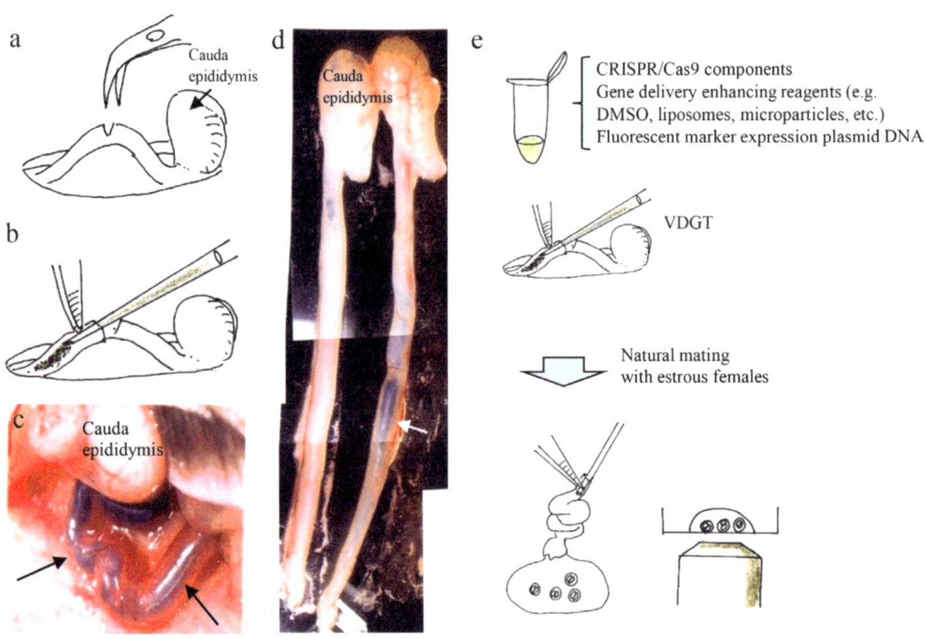

Figure 6.
Procedure for VDGT-based genome editing. (a–d) Experimental procedure of VDGT when TB as a visible marker is injected into the lumen of vas deferens. Under anesthesia, a small slit is made at the proximal region of vas deferens using micro scissors (a). Then, a glass micropipette is inserted into the lumen of vas deferens under observation using a dissecting microscope and the solution is slowly injected (b). After TB injection, the injected TB still remains within the proximal portion of vas deferens (arrows in c). One day after VDGT, the injected TB moves to the distal portion of vas deferens (arrow in d), showing the flow of the injected substance. e. Experimental procedure of VDGT when genome-editing components are injected into the lumen of vas deferens. First, a solution containing CRISPR/Cas9 components, gene delivery enhancing reagents (such as DMSO, liposomes, microparticles, etc.), and fluorescent marker expression plasmid DNA is prepared in a tube. Then, about 15 μL of this solution is immediately injected into the lumen of vas deferens. On the night following the VDGT or the next day, the VDGT-treated males are mated to normal estrous females. Later, cleavage stage embryos are collected to examine the presence/expression of the transgene (plasmid), as well as possible mutations in a target locus.

After short incubation period, this solution is injected into the lumen of vas deferens. Then, the VDGT-treated males are mated to normal estrous females on the day (night) or next day. Later, cleavage stage embryos were collected from the VDGT-treated females to examine the presence and expression of the transgene (plasmid) (**Figure 6e**, bottom) and occurrence of mutations in a target locus. In some cases, the SMGT-AI-treated females were allowed to deliver their pups to see whether genome editing is induced in their chromosomes.

6.2 SMGT-AI-based genome editing

AI is one of the assisted reproduction technologies that is based on the introduction of isolated sperm into the female reproductive tracts, such as uterine horn or oviductal lumen, to *in vivo* fertilize ovulated oocytes. As previously described in Section 3, isolated sperm are incubated in a solution containing exogenous DNA and gene delivery enhancing reagents such as DMSO, liposomes, and microparticles, for a short period (SMGT), and then the transfected sperm are subjected to AI, called "SMGT-based AI" (SMGT-AI). During this process, the exogenous DNA should be transmitted to oocytes via fertilization resulting in Tg embryos.

We previously reported that transfer of sperm into a space near the infundibulum between the ovary and ovarian bursa enables *in vivo* fertilization of ovulated oocytes in the ampulla region of the oviduct [133, 134]. In more detail, 2 μL of fresh epididymal B6C3F1 (F1 hybrid mice between C57BL/6 and C3H) sperm (containing 2 x 10^5 spermatozoa) were intrabursally injected 7 h after human chorionic gonadotropin (hCG) administration to B6C3F1 females that had been administrated with pregnant mare serum gonadotropin (PMSG) 48 h before. At 1.7 days after AI, normal cleaving embryos were recovered at rates of 40–100%. We called this AI technology "intrabursal transfer of sperm" (ITS) [133]. In **Figure 7a**, the ITS procedure is schematically illustrated. In **Figure 7b** and **c**, photographs before (b) and after (c) ITS are shown by using TB as a dye to visualize the process of AI. It is clear that the injected solution is present between the ovary and ovarian bursa (arrow in **Figure 7c**). In **Figure 7d**, an example for SGMT-AI-mediated genome editing in embryos is schematically shown. First, sperm isolated from the vas deferens are treated with CRISPR/Cas9 components (sgRNA + DNA/mRNA/protein for Cas9), gene delivery enhancing reagents (such as DMSO, liposomes, microparticles, etc.), and fluorescent marker expression plasmid DNA for a short period. Then, the solution containing the transfected sperm is subjected to AI towards females 7 h after hCG administration. The next day, 2-cell embryos are collected from the AI-treated females to examine the presence and expression of the transgene (plasmid) and occurrence of mutations in a target locus. In some cases, the SMGT-AI-treated females are allowed to deliver their pups to see whether genome editing is induced in their chromosomes. Notably, the selection of a successfully genome-edited sperm prior to AI may accelerate the production efficiency of genome edited offspring, although the practical approach for this remains unknown at present. Therefore, the success or failure of genome editing performed in this system may depend on the molecular analysis of the offspring (e.g. blastocysts or fetuses) generated after AI of the SMGT-treated sperm.

7. Conclusion

TMGT, based on direct *in vivo* gene delivery towards interstitial space of a testis, ST within a testis, or excurrent ducts of epididymides and vas deferens, is less labor

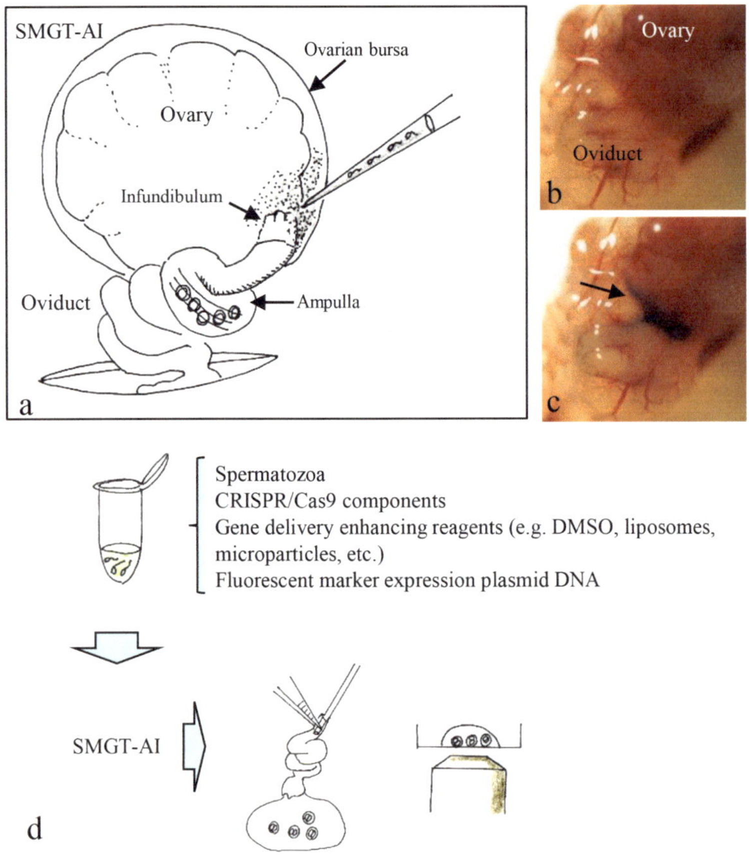

Figure 7.
Procedure for SMGT-AI-based genome editing. (a) ITS procedure schematic. (b, c) Photographs during before (b) and after (c) ITS, which is shown by intrabursal injection of TB. Note the presence of TB between the ovary and ovarian bursa (arrow in c). (d) Experimental procedure of SMGT-AI when genome-editing components are injected between the ovary and ovarian bursa. First, sperm isolated from the vas deferens are incubated in a solution containing CRISPR/Cas9 components, gene delivery enhancing reagents (such as DMSO, liposomes, microparticles, etc.) and fluorescent marker expression plasmid DNA for a short period. Then, the solution containing the transfected sperm is subjected to AI towards females 7 h after hCG administration. Later, cleavage stage embryos are collected to examine the presence/expression of the transgene (plasmid), as well as possible mutations in a target locus.

intensive and less time consuming for the production of GM animals. This testicular route is also ethically superior since fewer mice are required than existing alternative methods of transgenesis. The TMGT-treated males can be used to mate with estrous females, through which the exogenous genetic materials are transferred to oocytes at fertilization. During this process, there is no need for *ex vivo* handling of embryos, which is strictly required for zygote-based gene modification such as microinjection, EP, viral infection, and TransICSI. SMGT-AI, based on AI of sperm that have been transfected *in vitro* with the exogenous DNA, is also a convenient system for production of Tg animals, like TMGT. The CRISPR/Cas9 system, one of the recently developed genome editing technologies, is now recognized as a powerful and simple tool to create GM animals. More importantly, in this system, chromosomal integration of the genome editing components is not the prerequisite. Coupling this genome editing system with TMGT or SMGT-AI would accelerate creation of genome-edited animals in a more convenient manner. Furthermore, TMGT/SMGT-AI will be particularly useful for other animals that are difficult to manipulate as early embryos *in vitro*.

Acknowledgements

This study was partly supported by a grant (no. 24580411 for M.S.; no. 16H05049 and 16 K15063 for S.N.) from the Ministry of Education, Science, Sports, and Culture, Japan.

Author Contributions: Masahiro Sato designed the study and drafted the manuscript; Shingo Nakamura critically revised the manuscript.

Conflicts of interest

The founding sponsors had no role in the design of the study, collection, analyses, or interpretation of data, writing of the manuscript, and decision to publish the results.

Author details

Masahiro Sato[1*] and Shingo Nakamura[2]

1 Section of Gene Expression Regulation, Frontier Science Research Center, Kagoshima University, Kagoshima, Japan

2 Division of Biomedical Engineering, National Defense Medical College Research Institute, Saitama, Japan

*Address all correspondence to: masasato@m.kufm.kagoshima-u.ac.jp

References

[1] Gama Sosa MA, De Gasperi R, Elder GA. Animal transgenesis: An overview. Brain Structure and Function. 2010;**214**:91-109. DOI: 10.1007/s00429-009-0230-8

[2] Miao X. Recent advances in the development of new transgenic animal technology. Cellular and Molecular Life Sciences. 2013;**70**:815-828. DOI: 10.1007/s00018-012-1081-7

[3] Gordon JW, Scangos GA, Plotkin DJ, Barbosa JA, Ruddle FH. Genetic transformation of mouse embryos by microinjection of purified DNA. Proceedings of the National Academy of Sciences of the United States of America. 1980;**77**:7380-7384. DOI: 10.1073/pnas.77.12.7380

[4] Dunn DA, Pinkert CA, Kooyman DL. Foundation review: Transgenic animals and their impact on the drug discovery industry. Drug Discovery Today. 2005;**10**:757-767. DOI: 10.1016/S1359-6446(05)03452-5

[5] Houdebine LM. Transgenic animal models in biomedical research. Methods in Molecular Biology. 2007;**360**:163-202. DOI: 10.1385/1-59745-165-7:163

[6] van der Putten H, Botteri FM, Miller AD, Rosenfeld MG, Fan H, et al. Efficient insertion of genes into the mouse germ line via retroviral vectors. Proceedings of the National Academy of Sciences of the United States of America. 1985;**82**:6148-6152. DOI: 10.1073/pnas.82.18.6148

[7] Lois C, Hong EJ, Pease S, Brown EJ, Baltimore D. Germline transmission and tissue specific expression of transgenes delivered by lentiviral vectors. Science. 2002;**295**:868-872. DOI: 10.1126/science.1067081

[8] Torres M. The use of embryonic stem cells for the genetic manipulation of the mouse. Current Topics in Developmental Biology. 1998;**36**:99-114. DOI: 10.1016/S0070-2153(08)60497-4

[9] Hadjantonakis A, Gertsenstein M, Ikawa M, Okabe M, Nagy A. Generating green fluorescent mice by germline transmission of green fluorescent ES cells. Mechanisms of Development. 1998;**76**:79-90. DOI: 10.1016/S0925-4773(98)00093-8

[10] Beard C, Hochedlinger K, Plath K, Wutz A, Jaenisch R. Efficient method to generate single-copy transgenic mice by site-specific integration in embryonic stem cells. Genesis. 2006;**44**:23-28. DOI: 10.1002/gene.20180

[11] Wilmut I, Schnieke AE, McWhir J, Kind AJ, Campbell KHS. Viable offspring derived from fetal and adult mammalian cells. Nature. 1997;**385**:810-813. DOI: 10.1038/385810a0

[12] Cibelli JB, Stice SL, Golueke PJ, Kane JJ, Jerry J, et al. Cloned transgenic calves produced from nonquiescent fetal fibroblasts. Science. 1998;**280**:1256-1258. DOI: 10.1126/science.280.5367.1256

[13] Baguisi A, Behboodi E, Melican DT, Pollock JS, Destrempes MM, et al. Production of goats by somatic cell nuclear transfer. Nature Biotechnology. 1999;**17**:456-461. DOI: 10.1038/8632

[14] Perry AC, Wakayama T, Kishikawa H, Kasai T, Okabe M, et al. Mammalian transgenesis by intracytoplasmic sperm injection. Science. 1999;**284**:1180-1183. DOI: 10.1126/science.284.5417.1180

[15] Chan AW, Luetjens CM, Dominko T, Ramalho-Santos J, Simerly CR, et al. Foreign DNA transmission by ICSI: Injection of spermatozoa bound with exogenous DNA results in embryonic GFP expression and live rhesus monkey births. Molecular Human Reproduction.

2000;**6**:26-33. DOI: 10.1093/molehr/6.1.26

[16] Takahashi G, Gurumurthy CB, Wada K, Miura H, Sato M, et al. GONAD: *G*enome-editing via *O*viductal *N*ucleic *A*cids *D*elivery system: A novel microinjection independent genome engineering method in mice. Scientific Reports. 2015;**5**:11406. DOI: 10.1038/srep11406

[17] Gurumurthy CB, Takahashi G, Wada K, Miura H, Sato M, et al. GONAD: A novel CRISPR/Cas9 genome editing method that does not require *ex vivo* handling of embryos. Current Protocols in Human Genetics. 2016;**88**:15.8.1-15.8.12. DOI: 10.1002/0471142905.hg1508s88

[18] Ohtsuka M, Sato M, Miura H, Takabayashi S, Matsuyama M, et al. *i*-GONAD: A robust method for in situ germline genome engineering using CRISPR nucleases. Genome Biology. 2018;**19**:25. DOI: 10.1186/s13059-018-1400-x

[19] Kobayashi T, Namba M, Koyano T, Fukushima M, Sato M, et al. Successful production of genome-edited rats by the rGONAD method. BMC Biotechnology. 2018;**18**:19. DOI: 10.1186/s12896-018-0430-5

[20] Takabayashi S, Aoshima T, Kabashima K, Aoto K, Ohtsuka M, et al. *i*-GONAD (improved genome-editing via oviductal nucleic acids delivery), a convenient *in vivo* tool to produce genome-edited rats. Scientific Reports. 2018;**8**:12059. DOI: 10.1038/s41598-018-30137-x

[21] Sato M, Ohtsuka M, Nakamura S. Intraoviductal instillation of a solution as an effective route for manipulating preimplantation mammalian embryos *in vivo*. In: Payan-Carreira R. (ed.) New Insights into Theriogenology. Rijeka: InTechOpen; 2018. p135-150. DOI:10.5772/intechopen.79106

[22] Lavitrano M, Camaioni A, Fazio VM, Dolci S, Farace MG, et al. Sperm cells as vectors for introducing foreign DNA into eggs: Genetic transformation of mice. Cell. 1989;**57**:717-723. DOI: 10.1016/0092-8674(89)90787-3

[23] Brinster RL, Sandgren EP, Behringer RR, Palmiter RD. No simple solution for making transgenic mice. Letters to the editor. Cell. 1989;**59**:239-241. DOI: 10.1016/0092-8674(89)90282-1

[24] Spadafora C. Sperm cells and foreign DNA: A controversial relation. BioEssays. 1998;**20**:955-964. DOI: 10.1002/(SICI)1521-1878(199811)20:11<955:AID-BIES11>3.0.CO;2-8

[25] Smith KR. Sperm cell mediated transgenesis: A review. Animal Biotechnology. 1999;**10**:1-13. DOI: 10.1080/10495399909525917

[26] Smith K, Spadafora C. Sperm-mediated gene transfer: Applications and implications. BioEssays. 2005;**27**:551-562. DOI: 10.1002/bies.20211

[27] Spadafora C. Sperm-mediated "reverse" gene transfer: A role of reverse transcriptase in the generation of new genetic information. Human Reproduction. 2008;**23**:735-740. DOI: 10.1093/humrep/dem425

[28] Smith KR, editor. Sperm-Mediated Gene Transfer: Concepts and Controversies. (Edited eBook). Sharjah: Bentham Science Publishers; 2012. DOI: 10.2174/97816080523701120101

[29] Shen W, Li L, Pan Q, Min L, Dong H, et al. Efficient and simple production of transgenic mice and rabbits using the new DMSO-sperm mediated exogenous DNA transfer method. Molecular Reproduction and Development. 2006;**73**:589-594. DOI: 10.1002/mrd.20401

[30] Kim TS, Lee SH, Gang GT, Lee YS, Kim SU, et al. Exogenous DNA uptake of boar spermatozoa by a magnetic nanoparticle vector system. Reproduction in Domestic Animals. 2010;**45**:e201-e206. DOI: 10.1111/j.1439-0531.2009.01516.x

[31] Sato M, Iwase R, Kasai K, Tada N. Direct injection of foreign DNA into mouse testis as a possible alternative of sperm-mediated gene transfer. Animal Biotechnology. 1994;**5**:19-31. DOI: 10.1080/10495399409525801

[32] Sato M, Gotoh K, Kimura M. Sperm-mediated gene transfer by direct injection of foreign DNA into mouse testis. Transgenics. 1999;**2**:357-369

[33] Sato M, Yabuki K, Watanabe T, Kimura M. Testis-mediated gene transfer (TMGT) in mice: Successful transmission of introduced DNA from F0 to F2 generations. Transgenics. 1999;**3**:11-22

[34] Ogawa S, Hayashi K, Tada N, Sato M, Kurihara T, et al. Gene expression in blastocysts following direct injection of DNA into testis. Journal of Reproduction and Development. 1995;**41**:379-382. DOI: 10.1262/jrd.41.379

[35] Blanchard KT, Boekelheide K. Adenovirus-mediated gene transfer to rat testis in vivo. Biology of Reproduction. 1997;**56**:495-500. DOI: 10.1095/biolreprod56.2.495

[36] Muramatsu T, Shibata O, Ryoki S, Ohmori Y, Okumura J. Foreign gene expression in the mouse testis by localized in vivo gene transfer. Biochemical and Biophysical Research Communications. 1997;**233**:45-49. DOI: 10.1016/S0305-0491(99)00148-0

[37] Chang K-T, Ikeda A, Hayashi K, Furuhata Y, Nishihara M, et al. Production of transgenic rats and mice by the testis-mediated gene transfer. Journal of Reproduction and Development. 1999;**45**:29-36. DOI: 10.1262/jrd.45.29

[38] Chang K-T, Ikeda A, Hayashi K, Furuhata Y, Banai M, et al. Possible mechanisms for the testis-mediated gene transfer as a new method for producing transgenic animals. Journal of Reproduction and Development. 1999;**45**:37-42. DOI: 10.1262/jrd.45.37

[39] Sato M, Watanabe T, Yasuoka Y, Kodama H, Kimura M. Testis-mediated gene transfer (TMGT) in mice: Attempts to improve TMGT using commercially available reagents used for gene transfer in mammalian culture system. Transgenics. 2001;**3**:131-141

[40] Yonezawa T, Furuhata Y, Hirabayashi K, Suzuki S, Takahashi M, et al. Detection of transgene in progeny at different developmental stages following testis-mediated gene transfer. Molecular Reproduction and Development. 2001;**60**:196-201. DOI: 10.1002/mrd.1077

[41] Ryoki S, Park H, Ohmori Y, Shoji-Tanaka A, Muramatsu T. An integrase facilitates long-lasting foreign gene expression in vivo in mouse spermatogenic cells. Journal of Bioscience and Bioengineering. 2001;**91**:363-367. DOI: 10.1016/S1389-1723(01)80152-3

[42] Sato M, Ishikawa A, Kimura M. Direct injection of foreign DNA into mouse testis as a possible in vivo gene transfer system via epididymal spermatozoa. Molecular Reproduction and Development. 2002;**61**:49-56. DOI: 10.1002/mrd.1130

[43] Mogas T, Fernández-Novell JM, Palomo MJ, Otaegui PJ, Gomis RR, et al. Expression of a green fluorescence protein-carrier protein into mouse spermatozoa. Biochemical and Biophysical Research Communications. 2002;**297**:841-846. DOI: 10.1016/S0006-291X(02)02295-7

[44] Lu JK, Fu BH, Wu JL, Chen TT. Production of transgenic silver sea bream (*Sparus sarba*) by different gene transfer methods. Marine Biotechnology. 2002;**4**:328-337. DOI: 10.1007/s10126-002-0027-8

[45] Widłak W, Scieglińska D, Vydra N, Małusecka E, Krawczyk Z. In vivo electroporation of the testis versus transgenic mice model in functional studies of spermatocyte-specific hst70 gene promoter: A comparative study. Molecular Reproduction and Development. 2003;**65**:382-388. DOI: 10.1002/mrd.10305

[46] Kojima Y, Sasaki S, Umemoto Y, Hashimoto Y, Hayashi Y, et al. Effects of adenovirus mediated gene transfer to mouse testis in vivo on spermatogenesis and next generation. Journal of Urology. 2003;**170**:2109-2114. DOI: 10.1097/01.ju.0000092898.91658.08

[47] Sato M, Nakamura S. Testis-mediated gene transfer (TMGT) in mice: Effects of repeated DNA injections on the efficiency of gene delivery and expression. Transgenics. 2004;**4**:101-119

[48] Sato M, Nakamura S. A novel gene transmission pattern of exogenous DNA in offspring obtained after testis-mediated gene transfer (TMGT). Transgenics. 2004;**4**:121-135

[49] Kubota H, Hayashi Y, Kubota Y, Coward K, Parrington J. Comparison of two methods of in vivo gene transfer by electroporation. Fertility and Sterility. 2005;**83**(Suppl 1):1310-1318. DOI: 10.1016/j.fertnstert.2004.12.029

[50] Umemoto Y, Sasaki S, Kojima Y, Kubota H, Kaneko T, et al. Gene transfer to mouse testes by electroporation and its influence on spermatogenesis. Journal of Andrology. 2005;**26**:264-271. DOI: 10.1002/j.1939-4640.2005.tb01094.x

[51] Lu L, Lin M, Xu M, Zhou ZM, Sha JH. Gene functional research using polyethylenimine-mediated in vivo gene transfection into mouse spermatogenic cells. Asian Journal of Andrology. 2006;**8**:53-59. DOI: 10.1111/j.1745-7262.2006.00089.x

[52] Chen HL, Yang HS, Huang R, Tsai HJ. Transfer of a foreign gene to Japanese abalone (*Haliotis diversicolor supertexta*) by direct testis-injection. Aquaculture. 2006;**253**:249-258. DOI: 10.1016/j.aquaculture.2005.09.017

[53] He X, Qi B, Liu G, Yu W, Chen Q. A novel method to transfer gene in vivo system. Progress in Biochemistry and Biophysics. 2006;**33**:685-690

[54] Dhup S, Majumdar SS. Transgenesis via permanent integration of genes in repopulating spermatogonial cells *in vivo*. Nature Methods. 2008;**5**:601-603. DOI: 10.1038/nmeth.1225

[55] Li B, Sun G, Sun H, Xu Q, Gao B, et al. Efficient generation of transgenic chickens using the spermatogonial stem cells in vivo and ex vivo transfection. Science in China Series C-Life Sciences. 2008;**51**:734-742. DOI: 10.1007/s11427-008-0100-2

[56] Liu L, Cao F, Cai K, Zhang Y, Ding Z, et al. Generation of sperms containing EGFP-LacZ following transfection of chicken testis with a eukaryotic dual reporter vector. Reproduction in Domestic Animals. 2010;**46**:e39-e45. DOI: 10.1111/j.1439-0531.2010.01625.x

[57] Amaral MG, Campos VF, Seixas FK, Cavalcanti PV, Selau LP, et al. Testis-mediated gene transfer in mice: comparison of transfection reagents regarding transgene transmission and testicular damage. Biological Research. 2011;**44**:229-234. DOI: / S0716-97602011000300003

[58] Miao XY, Zhang X. Production of transgenic mice carrying the Thanatin gene by intratesticular injection. Biochemical and Biophysical Research

Communications. 2011;**415**:429-433. DOI: 10.1016/j.bbrc.2011.10.044

[59] Hui-ming JU, Li-jing BAI, Hong-yan REN, Yu-lian MU, Shu-lin YANG, et al. Production of transgenic mice by type-A spermatogonia-mediated gene transfer. Agricultural Sciences in China. 2011;**10**:431-437. DOI: 10.1016/S1671-2927(11)60022-9

[60] Usmani A, Ganguli N, Sarkar H, Dhup S, Batta SR, et al. A nonsurgical approach for male germ cell mediated gene transmission through transgenesis. Scientific Reports. 2013;**3**:3430. DOI: 10.1038/srep03430

[61] Chen H, Yin Y, Zhang Y, Sun M, Chen T, et al. Production of transgenic mice expressing the goat H-FABP gene by intratesticular injection. Molecular Biology Reports. 2013;**40**:2215-2222. DOI: 10.1007/s11033-012-2283-7

[62] Chen X, Zhang Z, Chang X, Niu Y, Cui H. Production of transgenic mice expressing tumor virus A under ovarian-specific promoter 1 control using testis-mediated gene transfer. Molecular Medicine Reports. 2014;**9**:955-960. DOI: 10.3892/mmr.2013.1876

[63] Raina A, Kumar S, Shrivastava R, Mitra A. Testis mediated gene transfer: in vitro transfection in goat testis by electroporation. Gene. 2015;**554**:96-100. DOI: 10.1016/j.gene.2014.10.030

[64] Pradhan BS, Majumdar SS. An efficient method for generation of transgenic rats avoiding embryo manipulation. Molecular Therapy—Nucleic Acids. 2016;**5**:e293. DOI: 10.1038/mtna.2016.9

[65] Usmani A, Ganguli N, Jain SK, Ganguli N, Sarkar RK, et al. Robust generation of transgenic mice by simple hypotonic solution mediated delivery of transgene in testicular germ cells. Molecular Therapy-Methods and Clinical Development. 2016;**3**:16076. DOI: 10.1038/mtm.2016.76

[66] Wang C, Sun G, Wang Y, Kong N, Chi Y, et al. Bacterial magnetic particles improve testes-mediated transgene efficiency in mice. Drug Delivery. 2017;**24**:651-659. DOI: 10.1080/10717544.2017.1293195

[67] Pramod RK, Mitra A. Intratesticular injection followed by electroporation allows gene transfer in caprine spermatogenic cells. Scientific Reports. 2018;**8**:3169. DOI: 10.1038/s41598-018-21558-9

[68] Kim JH, Jung-Ha HS, Lee HT, Chung KS. Development of a positive method for male stem cell-mediated gene transfer in mouse and pig. Molecular Reproduction and Development. 1997;**46**:515-526. DOI: 10.1002/(SICI)1098-2795(199704)46:4<515:AID-MRD10>3.0.CO;2-V

[69] Yamazaki Y, Fujimoto H, Ando H, Ohyama T, Hirota Y, et al. In vivo gene transfer to mouse spermatogenic cells by deoxyribonucleic acid injection into seminiferous tubules and subsequent electroporation. Biology of Reproduction. 1998;**59**:1439-1444. DOI: 10.1095/biolreprod59.6.1439

[70] Yamazaki Y, Yagi T, Ozaki T, Imoto K. In vivo gene transfer to mouse spermatogenic cells using green fluorescent protein as a marker. Journal of Experimental Zoology. 2000;**286**:212-218

[71] Huang Z, Tamura M, Sakurai T, Chuma S, Saito T, et al. In vivo transfection of testicular germ cells and transgenesis by using the mitochondrially localized jellyfish fluorescent protein gene. FEBS Letters. 2000;**487**:248-251. DOI: 10.1016/S0014-5793(00)02271-7

[72] Ikawa M, Tergaonkar V, Ogura A, Ogonuki N, Inoue K, et al. Restoration

of spermatogenesis by lentiviral gene transfer: Offspring from infertile mice. Proceedings of the National Academy of Sciences of the United States of America. 2002;**99**:7524-7529. DOI: 10.1073/pnas.072207299

[73] Yomogida K, Yagura Y, Nishimune Y. Electroporated transgene-rescued spermatogenesis in infertile mutant mice with a sertoli cell defect. Biology of Reproduction. 2002;**67**:712-717. DOI: 10.1095/biolreprod.101.001743

[74] Celebi C, Auvray P, Benvegnu T, Plusquellec D, Jegou B, et al. Transient transmission of a transgene in mouse offspring following in vivo transfection of male germ cells. Molecular Reproduction and Development. 2002;**62**:477-482. DOI: 10.1002/mrd.10143

[75] Kanatsu-Shinohara M, Toyokuni S, Shinohara T. Transgenic mice produced by retroviral transduction of male germ line stem cells in vivo. Biology of Reproduction. 2004;**71**:1202-1207. DOI: 10.1095/biolreprod.104.031294

[76] Ike A, Ohta H, Onishi M, Iguchi N, Nishimune Y, et al. Transient expression analysis of the mouse ornithine decarboxylase antizyme haploid-specific promoter using in vivo electroporation. FEBS Letters. 2004;**559**:159-164. DOI: 10.1016/S0014-5793(04)00065-1

[77] Hibbit O, Coward K, Kubota H, Prathalingham N, Holt W, et al. In vivo gene transfer by electroporation allows expression of a fluorescent transgene in hamster testis and epididymal sperm and has no adverse effects upon testicular integrity or sperm quality. Biology of Reproduction. 2006;**74**:95-101. DOI: 10.1095/biolreprod.105.042267

[78] Coward K, Kubota H, Hibbitt O, McIlhinney J, Kohri K, et al. Expression of a fluorescent recombinant form of sperm protein phospholipase C zeta in mouse epididymal sperm by in vivo gene transfer into the testis. Fertility and Sterility. 2006;**85**(Suppl 1):1281-1289. DOI: 10.1016/j.fertnstert.2005.12.012

[79] Parrington J, Coward K, Hibbitt O, Kubota H, Young C, et al. In vivo gene transfer into the testis by electroporation and viral infection - a novel way to study testis and sperm function. The Society for Reproduction and Fertility. 2007;**65**(Suppl):469-474

[80] Gonzalez-Gonzalez E, Lopez-Casas PP, Del MJ. Gene silencing by RNAi in mouse Sertoli cells. Reproductive Biology and Endocrinology. 2008;**6**:29. DOI: 10.1186/1477-7827-6-29

[81] Tang H, Kung A, Goldberg E. Regulation of murine lactate dehydrogenase C (Ldhc) gene expression. Biology of Reproduction. 2008;**78**:455-461. DOI: 10.1095/biolreprod.107.064964

[82] Hooley RP, Paterson M, Brown P, Kerr K, Saunders PTK. Intra-testicular injection of adenoviral constructs results in Sertoli cell-specific gene expression and disruption of the seminiferous epithelium. Reproduction. 2009;**137**:361-370. DOI: 10.1530/REP-08-0247

[83] Sehgal L, Thorat R, Khapare N, Mukhopadhaya A, Sawant M, et al. Lentiviral mediated transgenesis by *in vivo* manipulation of spermatogonial stem cells. PLoS One. 2011;**6**:e21975. DOI: 10.1371/journal.pone.0021975

[84] Li X, Mao Z, Wu M, Xia J. Rescuing infertility of *Pick1* knockout mice by generating testis-specific transgenic mice via testicular infection. Scientific Reports. 2013;**3**:2842. DOI: 10.1038/srep02842

[85] Kirby JL, Yang L, Labus JC, Lye RJ, Hsia N, et al. Characterization of epididymal epithelial cells-specific gene promoters by in vivo electroporation.

Biology of Reproduction. 2004;**71**:613-619. DOI: 10.1095/biolreprod.103.025635

[86] Esponda P, Carballada R. In-vivo gene transfer induces transgene expression in cells and secretions of the mouse cauda epididymis. Molecular Human Reproduction. 2009;**15**:355-361. DOI: 10.1093/molehr/gap026

[87] Huguet E, Esponda P. Foreign DNA introduced into the vas deferens is gained by mammalian spermatozoa. Molecular Reproduction and Development. 1998;**51**:42-52. DOI: 10.1002/(SICI)1098-2795(199809)51:1<42::AID-MRD5>3.0.CO;2-W

[88] Huguet E, Esponda P. Generation of genetically modified mice by spermatozoa transfection in vivo: Preliminary results. Molecular Reproduction and Development. 2000;**56**(2 Suppl):243-247. DOI: 10.1002/(SICI)1098-2795(200006)56:2+<243:AID-MRD6>3.0.CO;2-C

[89] Valenzuela M, Relloso M, Esponda P. In vivo transfection of the mouse vas deferens. Journal of Experimental Zoology. 2002;**293**:532-540. DOI: 10.1002/jez.90006

[90] Coward K, Kubota H, Parrington J. In vivo gene transfer into testis and sperm: Developments and future application. Archives of Andrology. 2007;**53**:187-197. DOI: 10.1080/01485010701426455

[91] Niu Y, Liang S. Progress in gene transfer by germ cells in mammals. Journal of Genetics and Genomics. 2008;**35**:701-714. DOI: 10.1016/S1673-8527(08)60225-8

[92] Parrington J, Coward K, Gadea J. Sperm and testis mediated DNA transfer as a means of gene therapy. Systems Biology in Reproductive Medicine. 2011;**57**:35-42. DOI: 10.3109/19396368.2010.514022

[93] Al-Shuhaib M, Al-Saadi A, Ewadh M, Noor M. Sperm mediated gene transfer in mammals; a versatile platform with multiple enhancements techniques. Journal of Biology, Agriculture and Healthcare. 2014;**4**:58-68

[94] Campos VF, Komninou ER, Urtiaga G, Leon PM, Seixas FK, et al. NanoSMGT: Transfection of exogenous DNA on sex-sorted bovine sperm using nanopolymer. Theriogenology. 2011;**75**:1476-1481. DOI: 10.1016/j.theriogenology.2011.01.009

[95] Campos VF, de Leon PMM, Komninou ER, Dellagostin OA, Deschamps JC, et al. NanoSMGT: Transgene transmission into bovine embryos using halloysite clay nanotubes or nanopolymer to improve transfection efficiency. Theriogenology. 2011;**76**:1552-1560. DOI: 10.1016/j.theriogenology.2011.06.027

[96] Barkalina N, Jones C, Kashir J, Coote S, Huang X, et al. Effects of mesoporous silica nanoparticles upon the function of mammalian sperm in vitro. Nanomedicine. 2014;**10**:859-870. DOI: 10.1016/j.nano.2013.10.011

[97] Wang Y, Zhao X, Du W, Liu J, Chen W, et al. Production of transgenic mice through sperm-mediated gene transfer using magnetic nano-carriers. Journal of Biomedical Nanotechnology. 2017;**13**:1673-1681. DOI: 10.1166/jbn.2017.2456

[98] Sperandio S, Lulli SV, Bacci ML, Forni M, Maione B, et al. Sperm-mediated DNA transfer in bovine and swine species. Animal Biotechnology. 1996;**7**:59-77. DOI: 10.1080/10495399609525848

[99] Yonezawa T, Furuhata Y, Hirabayashi K, Suzuki M, Yamanouchi K, et al. Protamine-derived synthetic peptide enhances the efficiency of sperm-mediated gene transfer using

liposome-peptide-DNA complex. Journal of Reproduction and Development. 2002;**48**:281-286. DOI: 10.1262/jrd.48.281

[100] Yang CC, Chang HS, Lin CJ, Hsu CC, Cheung JI, et al. Cock spermatozoa serve as the gene vector for generation of transgenic chicken (Gallus gallus). Asian-Australasian Journal of Animal Sciences. 2004;**17**:885-891. DOI: 10.5713/ajas.2004.885

[101] Harel-Markowitz E, Gurevich M, Shore LS, Katz A, Stram Y, et al. Use of sperm plasmid DNA lipofection combined with REMI (restriction enzyme-mediated insertion) for production of transgenic chickens expressing eGFP (enhanced green fluorescent protein) or human follicle-stimulating hormone. Biology of Reproduction. 2009;**80**:1046-1052. DOI: 10.1095/biolreprod.108.070375

[102] Schiestl RH, Petes TD. Integration of DNA fragments by illegitimate recombination in Saccharomyces cerevisiae. Proceedings of the National Academy of Sciences of the United States of America. 1991;**88**:7585-7589. DOI: 10.1073/pnas.88.17.7585

[103] Kuspa A. Restriction enzyme-mediated integration (REMI) mutagenesis. Methods in Molecular Biology. 2006;**346**:201-209. DOI: 10.1385/1-59745-144-4:201

[104] Collares T, Campos VF, de Leon PMM, Cavalcanti PV, Amaral MG, et al. Transgene transmission in chickens by sperm-mediated gene transfer after seminal plasma removal and exogenous DNA treated with dimethylsulfoxide or N,N-dimethylacetamide. Journal of Biosciences. 2011;**36**:613-620. DOI: 10.1007/s12038-011-9098-x

[105] Chaparian S, Abdulahnejad A, Rashidi F, Toghyani M, Gheisari A, et al. Is passive transmission of non-viral vectors through artificial insemination of sperm-DNA mixtures sufficient for chicken transgenesis? Journal of Reproduction and Development. 2016;**62**:265-270. DOI: 10.1262/jrd.2015-176

[106] Sun D, Zhuang X, Xiang X, Liu Y, Zhang S, et al. A novel nanoparticle drug delivery system: The anti-inflammatory activity of curcumin is enhanced when encapsulated in exosomes. Molecular Therapy. 2010;**18**:1606-1614. DOI: 10.1038/mt.2010.105

[107] de la Torre GC, Gorcham RV, Bech Serra JJ, Nann T, Kussmann M. “Exosomics”—A review of biophysics, biology and biochemistry of exosomes with a focus on human breast milk. Frontiers in Genetics. 2018;**9**:92. DOI: 10.3389/fgene.2018.00092

[108] Valadi H, Ekstrom K, Bossios A, Sjostrand M, Lee JJ, et al. Exosome-mediated transfer of mRNAs and microRNAs is a novel mechanism of genetic exchange between cells. Nature Cell Biology. 2007;**9**:654-659. DOI: 10.1038/ncb1596

[109] Vojtech L, Woo S, Hughes S, Levy C, Ballweber L, et al. Exosomes in human semen carry a distinctive repertoire of small non-coding RNAs with potential regulatory functions. Nucleic Acids Research. 2014;**42**:7290-7304. DOI: 10.1093/nar/gku347

[110] Sullivan R, Saez F, Girouard J, Frenette G. Role of exosomes in sperm maturation during the transit along the male reproductive tract. Blood Cells, Molecules and Diseases. 2005;**35**:1-10. DOI: 10.1016/j.bcmd.2005.03.005

[111] Hamatani T. Human spermatozoal RNAs. Fertility and Sterility. 2012;**97**:275-281. DOI: 10.1016/j.fertnstert.2011.12.035

[112] Ostermeier GC, Miller D, Huntriss JD, Diamond MP, Krawetz SA.

Reproductive biology: Delivering spermatozoan RNA to the oocyte. Nature. 2004;**429**:154. DOI: 10.1038/429154a

[113] Rassoulzadegan M, Grandjean V, Gounon P, Vincent S, Gillot I, et al. RNA-mediated non-Mendelian inheritance of an epigenetic change in the mouse. Nature. 2006;**441**:469-474. DOI: 10.1038/nature04674

[114] Wagner KD, Wagner N, Ghanbarian H, Grandjean V, Gounon P, et al. RNA induction and inheritance of epigenetic cardiac hypertrophy in the mouse. Developmental Cell. 2008;**14**:962-969. DOI: 10.1016/j.devcel.2008.03.009

[115] Grandjean V, Gounon P, Wagner N, Martin L, Wagner KD, et al. The miR-124-Sox9 paramutation: RNA-mediated epigenetic control of embryonic and adult growth. Development. 2009;**136**:3647-3655. DOI: 10.1242/dev.041061

[116] Cossetti C, Lugini L, Astrologo L, Saggio I, Fais S, et al. Soma-to-germline transmission of RNA in mice xenografted with human tumour cells: Possible transport by exosomes. PLoS One. 2014;**9**:e101629. DOI: 10.1371/journal.pone.0101629

[117] Jiang XC, Gao JQ. Exosomes as novel bio-carriers for gene and drug delivery. International Journal of Pharmaceutics. 2017;**521**:167-175. DOI: 10.1016/j.ijpharm.2017.02.038

[118] Alvarez-Erviti L, Seow Y, Yin HF, Betts C, Lakhal S, Wood MJA. Delivery of siRNA to the mouse brain by systemic injection of targeted exosomes. Nature Biotechnology. 2011;**29**:341-345. DOI: 10.1038/nbt.1807

[119] Lin Y, Wu J, Gu W, Huang Y, Tong Z, et al. Exosome-liposome hybrid nanoparticles deliver CRISPR/Cas9 system in MSCs. Advanced science (Weinheim, Baden-Württemberg, Germany). 2018;**5**:1700611. DOI: 10.1002/advs.201700611

[120] Horvath P, Barrangou R. CRISPR/Cas, the immune system of bacteria and archaea. Science. 2010;**327**:167-170. DOI: 10.1126/science.1179555

[121] Jinek M, Chylinski K, Fonfara I, Hauer M, Doudna JA, et al. A programmable dual-RNA-guided DNA endonuclease in adaptive bacterial immunity. Science. 2012;**337**:816-821. DOI: 10.1126/science.1225829

[122] Hsu PD, Lander ES, Zhang F. Development and applications of CRISPR-Cas9 for genome engineering. Cell. 2014;**157**:1262-1378. DOI: 10.1016/j.cell.2014.05.010

[123] Peng R, Lin G, Li J. Potential pitfalls of CRISPR/Cas9-mediated genome editing. FEBS Journal. 2016;**283**:1218-1231. DOI: 10.1111/febs.13586

[124] Ryu J, Prather RS, Lee K. Use of gene-editing technology to introduce targeted modifications in pigs. Journal of Animal Science and Biotechnology. 2018;**9**:5. DOI: 10.1186/s40104-017-0228-7

[125] Sonoda E, Hochegger H, Saberi A, Taniguchi Y, Takeda S. Differential usage of non-homologous end-joining and homologous recombination in double strand break repair. DNA Repair. 2006;**5**:1021-1029. DOI: 10.1016/j.dnarep.2006.05.022

[126] Chen K, Gao C. Targeted genome modification technologies and their applications in crop improvements. Plant Cell Reports. 2014;**33**:575-583. DOI: 10.1007/s00299-013-1539-6

[127] Kim YG, Cha J, Chandrasegaran S. Hybrid restriction enzymes: Zinc finger fusions to Fok I cleavage domain. Proceedings of the National Academy

of Sciences of the United States of America. 1996;**93**:1156-1160. DOI: 10.1073/pnas.93.3.1156

[128] Urnov FD, Miller JC, Lee YL, Beausejour CM, Rock JM, et al. Highly efficient endogenous human gene correction using designed zinc-finger nucleases. Nature. 2005;**435**:646-651. DOI: 10.1038/nature03556

[129] Sato M, Ohtsuka M, Watanabe W, Gurumurthy CB. Nucleic acids delivery methods for genome editing in zygotes and embryos: The old, the new, and the old-new. Biology Direct. 2016;**11**:16. DOI: 10.1186/s13062-016-0115-8

[130] Ran FA, Hsu PD, Lin CY, Gootenberg JS, Konermann S, et al. Double nicking by RNA-guided CRISPR Cas9 for enhanced genome editing specificity. Cell. 2013;**154**:1380-1389. DOI: 10.1016/j.cell.2013.08.021

[131] Kim S, Kim D, Cho SW, Kim J, Kim JS. Highly efficient RNA-guided genome editing in human cells via delivery of purified Cas9 ribonucleoproteins. Genome Research. 2014;**24**:1012-1019. DOI: 10.1101/gr.171322.113

[132] Guilinger JP, Thompson DB, Liu DR. Fusion of catalytically inactive Cas9 to FokI nuclease improves the specificity of genome modification. Nature Biotechnology. 2014;**32**:577-582. DOI: 10.1038/nbt.2909

[133] Sato M, Kimura M. Intrabursal transfer of spermatozoa (ITS): A new route for artificial insemination of mice. Theriogenology. 2001;**55**:1881-1890. DOI: 10.1016/S0093-691X(01)00529-5

[134] Sato M, Tanigawa M, Watanabe T. Effect of time of ovulation on fertilization after intrabursal transfer of spermatozoa (ITS): Improvement of a new method for artificial insemination in mice. Theriogenology. 2004;**62**:1417-1429. DOI: 10.1016/j.theriogenology.2004.02.018

Section 3

Genetically Modified Organism (GMO)

Chapter 4

Molecular Identification of Genetically Modified Crops for Biosafety and Legitimacy of Transgenes

Shahid Nazir, Muhammad Zaffar Iqbal and Sajid-ur-Rahman

Abstract

Crops undergo artificially DNA modifications for improvements are considered as genetically modified (GM) crops. These modifications could be in indigenous DNA or by introduction of foreign DNA as transgenes. There are 29 different crops and fruit trees in 42 countries, which have been successfully modified for various traits like herbicide tolerance, insect/pest resistance, disease resistance and quality improvement. GM crops are grown worldwide and its area is significantly increasing every year. Many countries have very strict rules and regulations for GM crops and are also a trade barrier in some situations. Hence, identification and testing of crops for GM contents is important for identity and legitimacy of transgene to simplify the international trade. Normally, molecular identification is performed at three different levels, i.e., DNA, RNA and protein, and each level has its own importance in testing about the nature and type of GM crops. In this chapter, current scenario of GM crops and different molecular testing tools are described in brief.

Keywords: biotechnology, genetic engineering, transgenic plants, molecular testing, polymerase chain reaction, enzymes linked Immuno-sorbent assay

1. Introduction

Biotechnology is a set of scientific tools in which living organisms are used for the welfare of mankind. This technique is efficiently used to modify and improve plants, animals and other microorganisms to increase their value. Biotechnology has a very wide range of applications and almost every field of daily science get benefit from this technology. Application of biotechnology in the field of agriculture has been practiced for a long time as people have wanted to improve agriculturally important crops by selection and breeding. In 1970s with the advancements in molecular biology, researchers were able to modify DNA which is a chemical building block and specify the features of living organisms at molecular level. This modification in genetic material or DNA is called as recombinant DNA technology or genetic engineering [1]. With the involvement of genetic engineering in agriculture, one can transfer useful hereditary/genetic information from distant sources into targeted crop which was not possible through traditional breeding methods. This genetic information is coded in the form of DNA or genes. Genes from any living organisms (human, animal, plant and microorganism) could be easily manipulated and transferred into other organisms to enhance their value. Organisms artificially modified at genome level using genetic engineering tools are termed as genetically modified organisms (GMOs). Microorganisms, i.e., bacteria and viruses have been genetically modified for the production of different kinds of medicines, pharmaceuticals and food ingredients [2]. Genetic engineering also has a great role in the field of agriculture by developing the transgenic crops for various traits. For example, a useful gene from bacteria, fungi and animals etc. could be isolated, cloned and integrated into desired crop to develop resistance against diseases and pests, drought and salinity tolerance or to improve the quality related traits etc. and are known GM crops [3]. After transformation, the transgenes replicate with indigenous plant genes and produce specific protein [4]. Biotechnology supports in practical exploitation of genetic material for the betterment of mankind. By using latest trends in genetic engineering one can create the new face of existing cultivars with improved and desirable characteristics. In addition to the improvement of agronomic traits, scientists are also looking in the production and expression of commercially valuable protein in plants like spider silk protein and polymers used in surgery [5]. A huge number of human vaccines, antigens and other pharmaceutical products are very efficiently expressing in transgenic plants. GMO offer many benefits to humans, but at the same time people also worry about the possible threats of using GMOs. These risks include the possible introduction of allergens in GM foods and transfer of selection marker genes which are normally antibiotic resistant genes to gut flora [6–8].

With the introduction of foreign genes, there are also some biosafety issues linked with GM crops. Such crops are often unintentionally or intentionally used for food and feed production. In some conditions, GM crops spread globally by trading, transportation and storage either intentionally or unintentionally and contaminate GM free items. Many countries have very strict rules and regulations for the development, cultivation, commercialization and labeling of GM crops and is also a trade barrier in some situations [9]. For example, USA has an optional labeling of GM in food items, whereas European Union has very strict rules for approval, cultivation and use of GM crops, including a compulsory labeling system [10]. They require very comprehensive information about such crops like type of targeted crop and transgene, safety for humans, environment, animals and effects on other related non-modified crops [11–13]. The increase in GM crop production has been coupled with an intricate and asynchronous international regulatory approval system, requiring identification and testing of food and agricultural products for the presence of GM content to simplify international trade. Molecular identification of GM crops confirms the identity and type of modified product at each stage and assures compliance with import for GM food and feed [14]. The testing of GM crops could be performed in open field or under controlled laboratory conditions that depends upon type of samples and sensitivity of test performed. Normally, molecular identification and testing of GM crops is performed at three different stages, i.e., DNA, RNA and protein. Each testing level has its own importance in testing the nature and type of GM crops. Generalized GM development methodology, global status, testing methods, possible biosafety issues and other benefits etc. are discussed in brief.

2. Global scenario of GM crops

The rapid acceptance of GM crops shows the significant benefits realized by large and small growers in both developed and under-developed countries growing GM crops commercially. Around 99% of global GM crops area is occupied by four major crops, i.e., soybean, maize, cotton and canola. USA is leading in the area under GM crops with 75.0 million hectares followed by Brazil and Argentina with 50.2 and 23.6 million hectares, respectively. In 2017, 24 countries planted 189.8

million hectares with an increase of 3.0% than 2016 [15]. Despite the possible health risks, cultivation area of GM crops is regularly increasing and introduction of new GM crops is continued. There are 29 different crops and fruit trees in 42, which countries have been successfully modified for various traits. A brief detail of GM crops, targeted/GM traits, number of GM events with responsible transgenes has been given in **Table 1**. Among GM trait distribution, herbicide

Sr. #	GM crops	GM events	GM traits	Transgenes
1	Alfalfa	05	Herbicide tolerant, Modified Product Quality	*cp4 epsps (aroA:CP4), ccomt (inverted repeat)*
2	Apple	03	Modified Product Quality	*PGAS PPO suppression gene*
3	Argentine Canola (*Brassica napus*)	41	Modified Product Quality, herbicide tolerant, Pollination control system	*te, gat4621, pat, cp4 epsps (aroA:CP4), goxv247, bar, barnase, barstar, phyA, bxn, Lackl-delta12D, Picpa-omega-3D, Micpu-delta-6D, Pyrco-delta-6E, Pavsa-delta-5D, Pyrco-delta-5E, Pavsa-delta-4D,*
4	Bean	01	Disease resistance	*ac1 (sense and antisense)*
5	Carnation	19	Herbicide tolerance , Modified flower color, Delayed ripening/senescence	*dfr, hfl (f3'5'h), surB, bp40 (f3'5'h), dfr-diaca, cytb5, acc (truncated)*
6	Flax	01	Herbicide tolerance	*als*
7	Maize	231	Male sterility , Fertility restoration , Modified alpha amylase , Herbicide tolerance, Insect resistance, Phytase production, Modified amino acid, Increased Ear Biomass, Drought stress tolerance,	*ms45, zm-aa1, amy797E, cry1Ab, pat, mepsps, mcry3A, ecry3.1Ab, cry1Fa2, cry1F, cry34Ab1, cry35Ab1, vip3Aa20, cp4 epsps (aroA:CP4), cry3Bb1, aad-1 , dam, zm-hra, gat4621 , vip3A(a), cry2Ab2, cry1A.105 , phyA2 , bar , cry9C, pinII, cry1Ac, 2mepsps , cordapA, goxv247,athb17 , dvsnf7, dmo, cspB, barnase, mocry1F epsps grg23ace5*
8	Cotton	60	Herbicide tolerance, insect resistance	*S4-HrA, pat, cry1Ac, cry1F, vip3A(a), aad-12, cp4 epsps (aroA:CP4), bar, bxn, cry2Ab2, cry2Ae, 2mepsps, cry1Ab-Ac cry1C, dmo, CpTI,*
9	Potato	48	insect resistance , Modified starch/carbohydrate, Reduced Acrylamide Potential , Reduced Black Spot, Viral disease resistance, Fungal Disease Resistance, Herbicide Tolerance	*cry3A, gbss (antisense fragment), asn1, ppo5, pvy_cp, plrv_orf1, plrv_orf2, cp4 epsps (aroA:CP4), Rpi-vnt1*
10	Linseed	01	herbicide tolerance	*als*
11	Eucalyptus	01	Volumetric Wood Increase	*cel1*
12	Eggplant	01	insect resistance	*Cry1Ac*
13	Creeping Bentgrass	01	Herbicide tolerance	*cp4 epsps (aroA:CP4)*
14	Chicory	03	Herbicide Tolerance, Male sterility	*bar, barnase*
15	Soybean	40	Modified Product Quality, Herbicide Tolerance, Insect resistance,	*gm-fad2-1 (silencing locus), pat, csr1-2, 2mepsps, aad-12, cp4 epsps (aroA:CP4), cry1Ac, cry1F, gm-fad2-1 (partial sequence), gat4601, gm-hra, hppdPF W336, Hahb-4, fatb1-A (sense and antisense segments), fad2-1A (sense and antisense), dmo, bbx32, cry1A.105, cry2Ab2, Pj.D6D, Nc.Fad3, avhppd-03, bar*
16	Poplar	02	Insect Resistance	*cry1Ac, API*
17	Plum	01	Viral disease resistance	*ppv_cp*
18	Petunia	01	Modified Product Quality	*chsA*
19	Papaya	02	Viral disease resistance	*prsv_rep, prsv_cp*
20	Melon	02	Delayed ripening/senescence	*sam-k*
21	Rose	02	Modified Product Quality	*5AT, bp40(f3'5'h)*
22	Rice	08	Modified Product Quality, Insect Resistance, Herbicide Tolerance	*crt1, psy1, 7crp,cry1Ab, cry1Ac, bar, cry1Ab (truncated)*
23	Squash	02	Viral disease resistance	*cmv_cp, zymv_cp, wmv_cp*
24	Sugar beet	03	Herbicide tolerance,	*cp4 epsps (aroA:CP4), goxv247, pat*
25	Sugarcane	04	Insect resistance, Drought stress tolerance	*cry1Ab, EcBetA, RmBetA*
26	Sweet pepper	01	Viral disease resistance	*cmv_cp*
27	Tobacco	01	Nicotine reduction	*NtQPT1 (antisense)*
28	Tomato	11	Delayed ripening/senescence , Insect resistance, Delayed fruit softening, Modified Product Quality, Viral disease resistance	*acc (truncated), sam-k, cry1Ac, accd, pg (sense or antisense), anti-efe, cmv_cp*
29	Wheat	01	Herbicide tolerant	*cp4 epsps (aroA:CP4)*

Table 1.
Summary of GM crops with modified traits and introduced transgenes.

tolerance (HT) enjoys the top position with 47% of the GM crops area. Stacked traits and insect resistance (IR) occupy 41 and 12% of the cultivated area of GM crops in 2017, respectively. The cultivation area under stacked traits, i.e., HT/IR is increasing very fast and various stacked gene products were got approved for food/feed and general commercialization. Soybean, maize and cotton are major crops developed with stacked traits [16]. Countries approving GM crops for food, feed and general cultivation are also increasing every year. In year 2017, 18 countries issued 176 approvals regarding GM crops cultivation, commercialization and use as food/feed [15].

3. GM crop's development methodology

Plants, in which one or more foreign genes are introduced artificially instead of plant getting them under natural conditions of cross-breeding or normal recombination, are known as GM plants. The introduced gene, known as transgene, could be from identical species or from different species within the same kingdom or other kingdom [17]. The process of introducing the transgene is called as genetic transformation that has become an important tool for crop improvement. Different steps are involved in the genetic transformation work like selection and identification of gene of interest (transgene), isolation from source organisms, cloning into suitable plasmid vector. Followed by development of expression vector containing all regulatory elements, i.e., promoters and terminators for regulation of transgene expression in targeted plants [18]. In addition, another gene cassette of selection is also the part of expression vector which serves as the primary selection of putative transgenic cells on artificial plant media. Normally two types of selection markers are used, antibiotic and visual selection markers, which depend upon the type of work. Final expression cassette is multiplied in suitable bacterial media and verified using various molecular biology techniques before transformation [19]. Integration of final expression cassette into plant can normally be achieved by two methods: (i) direct DNA delivery system, i.e., using biolistic gene gun by coating DNA on gold or tungsten particles and shooting on plant tissue with a specific pressure of helium gas (ii) introduction of gene by using biological vectors like disarmed Ti-plasmid of *Agrobacterium tumefaciens*. Both methods have successfully been used for the introduction of transgenes in plants [20]. Following genetic transformation, the transformed tissues are initially screened for transgene integration using selective plant tissue culture media. The regenerated plantlets on selective media supposed to have the transgenes and called as putative transgenics. Because there are three possibilities that the developed plantlets may be (i)

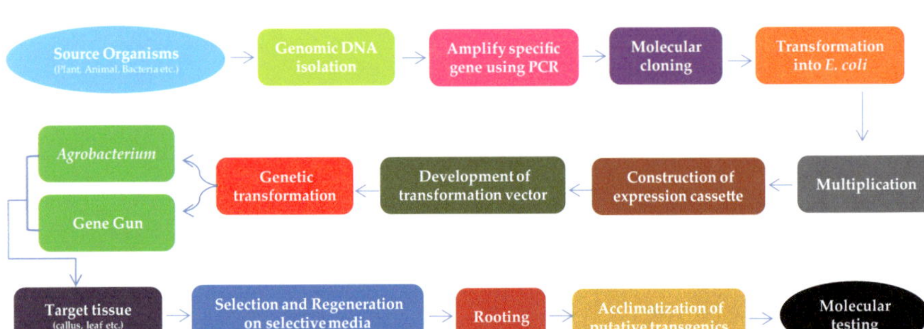

Figure 1.
General methodology for the development of genetically modified (GM) plants.

true transgenics (ii) escapees (iii) mutants. Hence, various molecular biological techniques like PCR, blotting, *E*nzyme-*l*inked *I*mmuno*S*orbent *A*ssay (ELISA) etc. are used to confirm transgene integration and true transgenics. The overall methodology for gene isolation, cloning, transformation and selection of putative transgenics has been shown in **Figure 1**.

4. Molecular test methods for the identification of GM crops

Introduction of GM crops and their products in markets required to be monitored and need to know the presence and type of GM elements. Labeling rules and trade requirements vary from country to country which necessitates for the development of reliable methods for the detection, identification and quantification of GM crop varieties and their products. GM crops can be tested by identifying either transgenes at DNA level, at transcriptional level by mRNA of transgene or using resulting trans-protein. There are many other methods like chromatography and mass spectrometry etc. which have their own importance in GMO testing. An overview of test methods used for detection and identification for GM crops has been given in **Figure 2**. Every test method has its own significance and value towards the final conclusion of GM crops. A brief summary of these methods has been shown in **Table 2**.

4.1 DNA based test methods

There are three main types of DNA based GMO testing methods.

4.1.1 Qualitative PCR

Polymerase Chain Reaction (PCR) is a primary method for screening of GM crops at DNA level. Qualitative analysis comprises of specific detection of target DNA sequence in test samples. Qualitative results clearly validate the presence or absence of GM elements under study, comparative to suitable controls and within the detection limits of analytical technique used, and test portion analyzed [21, 22]. This method has found very broad and wide applications in GMO detection as commonly accepted tool for regulatory purposes. In this method target gene/GM element multiplied to millions or billions by using gene specific primers. PCR process is basically comprised on three main steps, i.e., denaturation, annealing and extension in one cycle. In first step the double stranded DNA is separated into two single strands, primers then identify their homologous sequence and are annealed to each strand in second step. Third and final step involves making two identical copies of original DNA strand by adding exact nucleotides with the help of DNA polymerase at an appropriate temperature. These cycles repeated normally 40–50 times which results in an exponential amplification of target DNA/gene. Amplification of target gene occur in-vitro through a reaction catalyzed by a DNA polymerase in the presence of oligonucleotide primers and deoxyribonucleoside triphosphates in a defined reaction buffer [23, 24]. This amplified DNA can be visualized by using gel electrophoresis techniques. The results of this method will be either positive or negative for specific GM elements.

There are four testing methods which includes (i) Target-taxon specific (ii) Screening (iii) Construct-specific and (iv) Event-specific, these methods are generally used for the detection and identification of GM crops using PCR. Selection of specific and suitable primers is the most critical step in GMO detection which depends upon the testing method used. Brief detail of qualitative PCR based testing methods is given below:

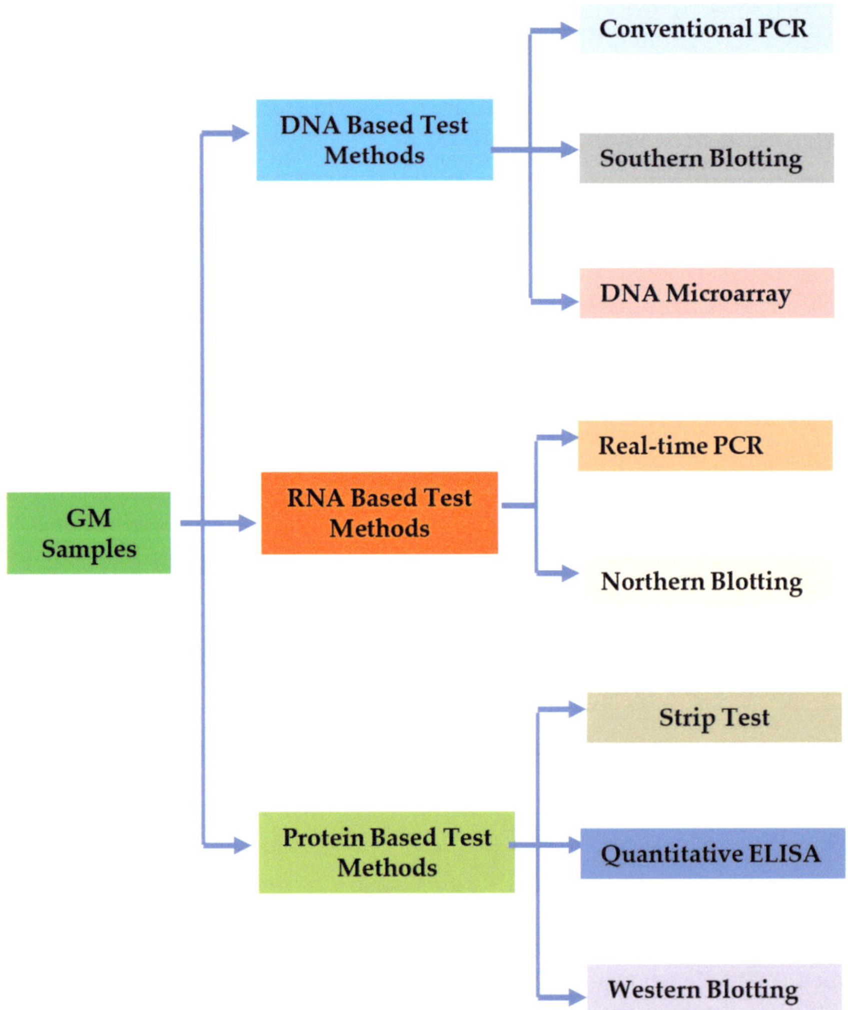

Figure 2.
Diagrammatic presentation of molecular test methods of GM crops.

4.1.1.1 Target-taxon specific method

PCR with various barcoding methods normally used for plant identification from mixed food samples particularly prepared from different plants. DNA barcode is broadly used technique for the detection and identification plants, animals or fungi texa by sequencing an optimized short DNA fragment. PCR and barcoding approaches identify specific texa very intelligently within samples of different origins [25–27]. This approach also plays very important role in the detection of mislabeled species and accidental or intentional species exchanges in food samples [28, 29]. The success of this method for identification and detection of species depends on the selected loci, because DNA barcode constitute a small portion of genome coupled with other PCR limiting factors, no single locus has been selected as universal DNA barcode region for all plant identification. For example lectin gene Le1 for soybean [30], chloroplast trnL intron for the identification of multicopy

Test methods	Test Name	Testing sample	Sensitivity /limit of detection	Conditions required	Advantages/ disadvantages
DNA based	Conventional PCR	DNA from Leaf/seed/processed food/feed items etc.	Highly sensitive/ 0.01%	Laboratory	Easy, broad range, used worldwide for GMO analysis
	Southern blotting		Highly sensitive		Require more time, sophisticated equipment/expertise, expensive, not used frequently
	DNA Microarray		Highly sensitive		
RNA based	Quantitative Real-time PCR	RNA converted in to cDNA before used in PCR	Highly sensitive	Laboratory	Broad range, allow actual quantification, require sophisticated equipment/expertise, expensive
	Northern blotting	RNA	Highly sensitive		Require more time, sophisticated equipment/expertise, expensive, not used frequently
Protein based	Strip test	Protein	Low sensitive/ 0.1-1.0%	May be perform in field	Easy, quick, cheap, not suitable for processed food
	Qualitative ELISA		Highly sensitive/ 0.01-0.1%	Laboratory	Not suitable for processed food, require expertise, expensive, results may vary from person-to-person and lab –to-lab of same sample
	Western blotting		Highly sensitive		Require more time, sophisticated equipment/expertise, expensive, not used frequently

Table 2.
Brief summary of GMO test methods.

DNA sequences in plants [31], polygalacturonase gene (PG gene) codes for a PG-enzyme that is linked with ripening in GM Zeneca tomato etc. [32].

4.1.1.2 Screening method

This is a most generalized method and widely used for the screening of GM crops from non-GM materials. This is not crop specific and can detect the GM elements even in raw and processed matrices like food and feed products developed from GM crops. In this method promoter, terminator and selection marker genes are the target elements in PCR. These are the bacterial gene sequences used to regulate the transgenes and selection of transgenic cells on artificial plant media [33, 34]. These genetic elements include cauliflower mosaic virus CaMV 35S promoter, *Agrobacterium tumifaciens* nopaline syhnthase NOS terminator and neomycin phosphotransferase NPTII etc. present in most commercialized GM crops in market. Hence, one can easily detect and identify the presence of GM crop by using specific primers of these genetic elements in PCR [35, 36].

4.1.1.3 Construct-specific method

In this method specific primer pairs normally got designed from the transformed gene construct. These construct could be transformed more than one crop for genetic improvement. The construct-specific detection method involves targeting the junction between two elements, and it is not able to distinguish two different events transformed with the same plasmid [37]. These methods either DNA or protein based. For practical reasons, several DNA sequences are shared by many GM crops and protein based methods detect the product of inserted DNA like Bt toxin in GM crops. Since different GM crops may produce the identical protein, this test method can detect a sample for several GMOs in one step. For examples GTS-40-3-2 GM construct for the development of roundup ready soybean, Zeneca F282 GM tomato, Bt11, Bt176 and T25 for GM maize etc.

4.1.1.4 Event-specific method

The junction sequences in the transgene integration points in the plant genome can be used to identify and detect the specific transformation event. The transgene integration site usually unique and specific for each transformation event due to lack of homologous recombination. Hence, different GM crops could be produced with similar gene construct and this event-specific detection method will be the only approach to differentiate between GM crops having similar transgenic cassette. This method can distinguish legitimate transgenic events from related unauthorized genotypes/varieties having identical transgene construct, thus this approach frequently used to assess the legality of GM crops [24]. Examples are Mon-531 event for Bollgard cotton, Mon-1445 event for Roundup Ready cotton, Mon-89,034 event for YieldGard VT Pro maize etc.

4.1.2 Southern blotting

Another DNA based GM crops identification techniques is southern blotting which was described by Southern in 1975 [38]. This test method is frequently used for the identification of specific DNA fragments transformed into the genome of transgenic plants or its products. This method could also be used in gene discovery and mapping, evolution and developmental studies, diagnostics and forensics etc. This test method involved five steps (i) DNA isolation and enzyme restriction (ii) electrophoresis for DNA separation (iii) shifting and fixing of separated DNA on suitable membrane (iv) hybridization with labeled probe and (v) detection by chemiluminescence or radioactive methods. This is very reliable method that provides the molecular evidence of the transgene integration and also estimates the copy number of introduced gene into the GMO genome. In comparison with PCR, this method associated with some limitations like it requires large amount of DNA, expensive, requires more time, proper infrastructure and trained manpower etc.

4.1.3 DNA microarray

A microarray is a laboratory method used to identify the expression of more than one gene in a single test. It is DNA based and new in comparison to previous protocols. This test method has been included in GMO screening as a method for simultaneous detection of more than 250,000 targets in single assay/chip [39–41]. This method consists of pre-amplification step of the desired targets, followed by hybridization on a chip having specific probes, and then detection step [42, 43]. So far, it is used for qualitative information of GMO, sometime semi-quantitative.

Use of microarray technology for the GMO detection is restrained as it require very special and costly equipment for scanning microarrays, chances of cross contamination and laborious in comparison with other techniques.

4.2 RNA based test methods

Transgenic DNA must be translated into protein to be an effective and have effects in an organism. This translation process occurs when DNA transcribed into messenger RNA (mRNA), and is considered as the intermediate step transferring information contained in DNA to protein. The presence of mRNA is directly associated with gene expression. Different molecular biology techniques used to monitor and study the gene expression in GMOs include real-time PCR, northern etc. These methods could be used to identify the transgene expression in various plant tissues and at different developmental phases in GMOs.

4.2.1 Quantitative real-time PCR

Gene expression normally verified in RT-PCR using isolated mRNA from GMOs. This test method is based on reverse transcription of mRNA and synthesis of complementary DNA (cDNA) which is then used as template in PCR amplification of target gene. The amplified fragment electrophoresed and visualized using agarose gel under UV. Intensity of amplified band in agarose gel give some indications of target mRNA in tested sample [44]. Quantitative RT-PCR is an up-to-date method, principally based on RT-PCR and is generally known as qRT-PCR. It is more robust, specific and sensitive, provides good quantitative results. The process of amplification is presented in real-time by capturing a fluorescent signal in more sophisticated way. In real-time assay of transgene in GMOs, the amplification and detection occur simultaneously [45].

4.2.2 Northern blotting

Similar to RT-PCR, northern blotting also requires mRNA as tested material from GMOs. This is a standard method for the analysis of size and level of target RNA in a complex GMO samples. Likewise southern blotting, it also composed on five steps, only difference is that the starting material is mRNA instead DNA and the labeled probe is complementary DNA (cDNA), which hybridizes the RNA. It gives comparative amount of gene expression at the RNA level. This is comparatively simple to perform, cheap and not overwhelmed by artifacts [46]. Recent advancements of hybridization membranes and buffers have resulted in increased sensitivity, closing the gap to the more laborious nuclease protection experiments. It is considered that this test method can study gene expression for a limited number of genes per analysis. This can be very useful to monitor the up- or down regulation of transgene for specific problem, but is not useful in monitoring the up- or down regulated genes are unknown.

4.3 Protein based test methods

Immunoassay protocols for the detection of GMOs by antibodies are the impressive for the detection of various types of proteins either qualitatively or quantitatively [47]. Two types of antibodies, i.e., monoclonal and polyclonal could be used depending on the need and specificity of detection method. Normally, *E*nzyme-*l*inked *I*mmuno*S*orbent *A*ssay (ELISA) and western blot methods have been used for the protein analysis in GMOs.

4.3.1 Qualitative strip test

Most common antibody based test for GMO screening is strip test method also known as lateral flow or dipstick test. It is qualitative in nature and gives the information about the presence or absence of specific proteins in tested samples. In this method, thin strip made-up of nitrocellulose membrane used which protected by a sample pad on one end and a wicking pad on other end. Test samples normally homogenized in suitable buffer solutions and membrane on strip wicks up the solution and it will move upward via capillary movement and protein will bind to its specific antibody. The results shown in the form of visible lines on the strip depicting that the specific protein is present in test sample. There are normally two lines appears on the strip, one for tested protein and second of control line showing the authenticity of all test procedure and strip used. The appearance of only control line on the strip, shows that sample is negative for transgenic protein, but the test was performed accurately [48]. This is very quick method to test GMOs which normally take 5–15 minutes to gives results [49]. In addition, it is cheap, easy to perform and not require specific equipment and special trained manpower. It can be performed in open field as well. Currently, strips are available to detect multiple proteins in single assay [50].

4.3.2 Quantitative ELISA test

Another more sensitive antibody-based protein identification method is *E*nzyme-*l*inked *I*mmuno*S*orbent *A*ssay (ELISA) also called a plate test or quantitative ELISA. It gives information about the quantity of protein in tested samples. In this assay protein specific antibody coated multi-well plate is used to identify and quantify the specific protein. Specific protein present will bind to antibody, following washing, another antibody specific for protein of interest and tagged with an enzyme is added to well [51]. The enzyme linked identification antibody will bind with specific protein and unbound antibody removed by washing. The color of the solution will change from blue to yellow by the addition of substrate for enzyme. Intensity of yellow color is directly proportional to amount of protein present in well. This GMO test method is more sensitive in comparison with strip test and can detect target protein even in very low concentrations. However, it requires more time, trained manpower and good laboratory facilities in contrast to strip test.

4.3.3 Western blotting

This is very specific method and provides the qualitative results of the target protein in GM crop sample. This method is very useful to analyze the insoluble proteins [47, 50]. Like other blotting techniques samples are solubilized with detergents and reducing agents and separated by electrophoresis and shifted to membrane. Binding immunoglobulin sites on membrane are blocked by dried nonfat milk and specific sites are probed with antibodies. Detection carried out using different staining agents silver nitrate of Coomassie, alkaline phosphatase etc. [18]. Its detection limit varies with test ample like 0.25% for seeds and 1.0% for toasted meal [52]. In comparison with other protein based assays, it is difficult method, and is capable of studying only a few samples at a time. Therefore, it is not frequently used in GMO testing activities but it is more used in research purpose to verify initial results generated by other testing method.

5. Certified/standard reference materials for GMO testing

Validity and authenticity of GMO testing results is doubtful until the use of positive and negative controls at each testing step. Use of certified reference material (CRM) or standard reference material (SRM) during testing produce not only validate the testing results but at the same time, assess the performance of test method, equipment, personnel and other environmental conditions in which testing being performed [52]. CRM must contain the certificate of analysis, should be prepared by following ISO-Guide 34, have information about which GM events or elements present and what is its concentration, storage requirements, preparation and expiry date etc. While SRM have all the similar information but lacks the certificate of analysis and was not prepared by a certified company. Bothe CRM and SRM could be used to validate the testing results but CRM is more reliable and globally acceptable. Each GMO needs specific CRM which is used in testing and conclusion about the presence of specific GM event/element in testing samples. Normally seeds of GM and Non-GM crops are mixed at specific percentage and homogenized to make powder before analysis [51]. The availability of CRM is presently restricted due to some concerns of IPR and expenses [53]. The Institute of Reference Materials and Measurements at the Joint Research Center (JRC) in Geel, Belgium, FAPAS Fera Science Ltd., Sand Hutton UK, American Oil Chemists Society (AOCS), Urbana, Illinois, USA etc. are authorized companies to paper and sale of CRMs for GMO testing.

6. Pros and cons of GM crops

The most common improvement by the introduction of GM crops is the increase in yield and quality. There are many yield limiting factors like insect/pest, diseases, drought, heat, salinity, rapidly changing climatic conditions etc. Conventional approaches like irrigations, sprays and use of fertilizers etc. done a great job but the problem was increasing day-by-day. By the introduction of recombinant DNA technology in agricultural sector, scientists successfully develop the new face of existing cultivars with improved and desirable traits. The GM technologies increase the opportunities for plant breeders to develop crops that are protected from climatic stresses and attacks of insects and diseases [54, 55]. The crops have been successfully modified for herbicide tolerant, insect/pest resistance, disease resistance, abiotic stress tolerance, micronutrient enrichment etc. Furthermore, this technology helping us to improve the nutritional quality, longer shelf life, foods that are more appealing to eat and easier to transport. Development of various biopharmaceuticals and expression of human therapeutic proteins in plants also a great contribution of GM technology to improve the human life [56].

On the other hand there are also some biosafety issues linked with the use of GM crops. Biosafety means the need to protect human and animal health from possible adverse effects of GM technology. There are some reports about the potential threats linked with the use of GMOs like risks of allergineicity, development of herbicide tolerant weeds and resistant insects, harms to non-target organisms, selection marker gene could induce antibiotic resistant and reduce the effectiveness of antibiotics to cure disease etc. [7, 57–58]. Turning on of certain genes due to the use of strong promoters and might be harmful in humans, effects on the nutritional profiling, transgene may flow from non-target crops/weeds etc. Biosafety is an essential to modern biotechnology and the adoption of biotech products requires to be balanced with acceptable biosafety safeguards. Participation of different stakeholders and dissemination of information and knowledge in public about GM products is much important to safe use of this technology.

7. National scenario of GM crops, biosafety, labeling and trade aspects

Agriculture sector of Pakistan plays a dominant role in the economy with 18.9% contribution in Gross Domestic Product (GDP) and engages 42.3% labour force. It is also a chief source of foreign exchange earnings and provide raw material for progress of other sectors [59]. Pakistan stands at seventh position among 26 countries growing GM crops, and insect resistant GM cotton of Mon-531 event is the only crop grown in the country with adoption reaching 2.9 million hectares of total 3.0 million hectares cotton crop area. Mon-531 is the only approved commercialized GM event in the country having insecticidal *Cry1Ac* gene of *Bacillus thurengiiensis* to control the lepidopteron insects. In 2015, US$398 million economic gain was estimated with the adoption of GM cotton [60]. Moreover, field trials of GM maize hybrids have successfully been conducted for single and stacked insect resistant (IR) and herbicide tolerances (HT) traits. For single HT trait, Monsanto event NK-603 was tested, while for stacked traits, i.e., IR/HT, Mon-89,034 x NK-603, TC-1507 x Mon-810 x NK-603 and TC-1507 x NK-603 were studied. These GM traits were officially approved for commercial cultivation by National Biosafety Committee in 2016. Field performance trials were completed as the part of regulatory requirements and varietal registration by Federal Seed Certification and Registration Committee of National Food Security and Research ministry [15]. In near future, GM maize having IR and HT traits will be grown by farmers, and it will be the second approved GM crop in the country.

Pakistan is signatory to World Trade Organization (WTO) and has sanctioned Convention on Biological Diversity (CBD) in 1994 and Cartagena Protocols in 2009. Different legislations under the Agreement of Trade Related Aspects of Intellectual Property Rights have been disseminated in the country. In addition, Pakistan Biosafety rules were designed in 2005, which are responsible for safe use of GM technology, manufacturing, import and storage of GMOs. Following these, National Biosafety Guidelines were developed in which the procedures to undertake all linked activities to GMO work were highlighted. These guidelines were framed in accordance with the recommendations of Food and Agriculture Organization (FAO), World Health Organization (WHO), United Nations Industrial Development Organization (UNIDO) and United Nations Environment Programme (UNEP). As per these guidelines the biosafety aspects of GMO work are monitored at three different levels, i.e., Institutional Biosafety Committee (IBC), Technical Advisory Committee (TAC) and National Biosafety Committee (NBC). The applications related to GMO work are submitted to IBC, and after thorough evaluation, the case is submitted to TAC for assessment and recommendations, while NBC is the final body to take further action regarding its approval or rejection. NBC is responsible to looks after the laboratory research, field studies, commercial release, imports, exports and sale/purchase of GMOs and their products [61].

Pakistan exports rice, cotton, fruits (oranges and mangoes), vegetables and fish to its neighboring states, Middle East and Central Asian countries. IR cotton of Mon-531 event is the only one GM crop officially approved for general cultivation in the country. Very comprehensive testing procedures are adopted to test and verify the status of approved events in the candidate cotton varieties. Around 49 universities and 07 research institutes are actively involved in the teaching and research related to the development and testing of GM crops in the country [62]. In Pakistan, Agricultural Biotechnology Research Institute (ABRI) at Ayub Agricultural Research Institute (AARI), Faisalabad and SGS Laboratories Karachi have GMO testing labs, which have been accredited by Pakistan National Accreditation Council

(PNAC) for ISO-17025. These labs are efficiently working on the testing and identification of GM crops and are equipped with state-of-the-art facilities needed for the detection, identification and quantification of GMOs. All crop seeds being imported from other countries are first tested for the presence and type of GM elements from these laboratories and then allowed for cultivation in the country. All the import and export activities are strictly monitored with reference to GMOs.

8. Conclusion

Testing of GM crops is important issue for the legitimacy, biosafety and regulatory purposes. The area under GM crops is increasing very rapidly and many new genes are being introduced in major crops. For the safety of humans, environment, animals and other related micro-flora, a comprehensive molecular testing of newly developed GMO is very important before commercial release. Regulatory processes for GM crops approval need comprehensive risk analysis for each case separately. The detection and identification of GMOs is also of great value in identifying the purity of sample, labeling food and trade reasons. Therefore, combined use of more than one testing methods would be advantageous for complete analysis, authenticity and biosafety assessment of GM samples.

Author details

Shahid Nazir*, Muhammad Zaffar Iqbal and Sajid-ur-Rahman
Agricultural Biotechnology Research Institute, Ayub Agricultural Research Institute (AARI), Faisalabad, Pakistan

*Address all correspondence to: shahidnazir97@yahoo.com

References

[1] Harlander SK. The evolution of modern agriculture and its future with biotechnology. Journal of the American College of Nutrition. 2002;**21**:161S-165S. DOI: 10.1080/07315724.2002.10719260

[2] Atherton KT. Safety assessment of genetically modified crops. Toxicology. 2002;**181**:421-426. DOI: 10.1016/S0300-483X(02)00485-7

[3] Glass S, Jessica F. Genetic modification Technology for nutrition and improving diets: An ethical perspective. Current Opinions in Biotechnology. 2017;**44**:46-51. DOI: 10.1016/j.copbio.2016.11.005

[4] Beyaz R, Selcen ED, Aycan M, Kayan M, Yıldız M. A novel method for high-frequency transgenic shoot regeneration via *Agrobacterium tumefaciens* in flax (*Linum usitatissimum* L.). Journal of Plant Biotechnology. 2016;**43**:240-247. DOI: 10.5010/JPB.2016.43.2.240

[5] Ma JKC, Drake PMW, Christou P. Genetic modification: The production of recombinant pharmaceutical proteins in plants. Nature Reviews Genetics. 2003;**4**:794-805. DOI: 10.1038/nrg1177

[6] Yaqoob A, Ahmad AS, Tahir RS, Rao AQ, Khan MAZ, Sana T, et al. Risk assessment of Bt crops on the non-target plant-associated insects and soil organisms. Journal of the Science of Food and Agriculture. 2016;**96**:2613-2619. DOI: 10.1002/jsfa.7661

[7] Mesnage R, Clair E, Gress S, Then C, Székács A, Séralini GE. Cytotoxicity on human cells of Cry1ab and Cry1ac Bt insecticidal toxins alone or with a glyphosate-based herbicide. Journal of Applied Toxicology. 2013;**33**:695-699. DOI: 10.1002/jat.2712

[8] Bawa AS, Anilakumar KR. Genetically modified foods: Safety, risks and public concerns—A review. Journal of Food Science and Technology. 2013;**50**:1035-1046. DOI: 10.1007/s13197-012-0899-1

[9] Smyth SJ. Genetically modified crops, regulatory delays, and international trade. Food and Energy Security. 2017;**6**:78-86. DOI: 10.1002/fes3.100

[10] Smart RD, Blum M, Wesseler J. Trends in approval times for genetically engineered crops in the United States and the European Union. Journal of Agricultural Economics. 2016;**68**:182-198. DOI: 10.1111/1477-9552.12171

[11] Lu H, Katherine AM, John CB. Messages promoting genetic modification of crops in the context of climate change: Evidence for psychological reactance. Appetite. 2017;**108**:104-116. DOI: 10.1016/j.appet.2016.09.026

[12] Baig S, Khan MZU, Nadeem Z, Ahmed S, Mushtaq AS. GM crops and their environmental risks: A mini overview. Fuuast Journal of Biology. 2017;**7**:193-198

[13] Klümper W, Matin QA. Meta-analysis of the impacts of genetically modified crops. PLoS One. 2014;**9**:e111629. DOI: 10.1371/journal.pone.0111629

[14] Miraglia M, Berdal K, Brera C, Corbisier P, Holst-jensen A, Kok E, et al. Detection and traceability of genetically modified organisms in the food production chain. Food and Chemical Toxicology. 2004;**42**:1157-1180. DOI: 10.1016/j.fct.2004.02.018

[15] ISAAA. Global Status of Commercialized Biotech/GM Crops in 2017: Biotech Crop Adoption Surges as Economic Benefits Accumulate in 22

Years. Ithaca, NY: ISAAA; 2017. ISAAA Brief No. 53

[16] Gressel J, Aaron JG, Micheal ODK. How well will stacked transgenic Pest/herbicide resistances delay pests from evolving resistance? Pest Management Science. 2017;**73**:22-34. DOI: 10.1002/ps.4425

[17] Tripathi L. Techniques for detecting genetically modified crops and products. African Journal of Biotechnology. 2005;**4**:1472-1479. DOI: 10.4314/ajfand.v4i13.71830

[18] Sambrook J, Russell DW. Molecular Cloning: A Laboratory Manual. New York: Cold Spring Harbor Laboratory Press, Cold Spring Harbor; 2001

[19] Brown TA. Gene Cloning and DNA Analysis: An Introduction. 7th ed. Chichester, West Sussex ; Hoboken, NJ: John Wiley and Sons Ltd; 2016

[20] Rao AQ, Allah B, Sarfraz K, Kamran S, Ahmad AS, Husnain T, et al. The myth of plant transformation. Biotechnology Advances. 2009;**27**:753-763. DOI: 10.1016/j.biotechadv.2009.04.028

[21] Vijayakumar KR, Martin A, Gowda LR, Prakash V. Detection of genetically modified soya and maize: Impact of heat processing. Food Chemistry. 2009;**117**:514-521. DOI: 10.1016/j.foodchem.2009.04.028

[22] Saiki RK, Scharf S, Faloona F, Mullis KB, Horn GT, Erlich HA, et al. Enzymatic amplification of ß-globin genomic sequences and restriction site analysis for diagnosis of sickle cell anemia. Science. 1985;**230**:1350-1354. DOI: 10.1126/science.2999980

[23] Mullis KB, Faloona FA. Specific synthesis of DNA in vitro via a polymerase-catalyzed reaction. Methods in Enzymology. 1987;**155**:335-350. DOI: 10.1016/0076-6879(87)55023-6

[24] Holst-Jensen A, Rønning SB, Løvseth A, Berdal KG. PCR technology for screening and quantification of genetically modified organisms (GMOs). Analytical and Bioanalytical Chemistry. 2003;**375**:985-993. DOI: 10.1007/s00216-003-1767-7

[25] Coghlan ML, Haile J, Houston J, Murray DC, White NE, Moolhuijzen P, et al. Deep sequencing of plant and animal DNA contained within traditional Chinese medicines reveals legality issues and health safety concerns. PLoS Genetics. 2012;**8**:e1002657. DOI: 10.1371/journal.pgen.1002657

[26] Newmaster SG, Meghan G, Dhivya S, Sathishkumar R, Subramanyam R. DNA barcoding detects contamination and substitution in north American herbal products. BMC Medicine. 2013;**11**:222. DOI: 10.1186/1741-7015-11-222

[27] Tillmar AO, Barbara DA, Jenny W, Gunilla H. A universal method for species identification of mammals utilizing next generation sequencing for the analysis of DNA mixtures. PLoS One. 2013;**8**:e83761. DOI: 10.1371/journal.pone.0083761

[28] Galimberti A, Fabrizio AM, Alessia L, Ilaria B, Silvia F, Maurizio C, et al. DNA barcoding as a new tool for food traceability. Food Research International. 2013;**50**:55-63. DOI: 10.1016/j.foodres.2012.09.036

[29] Ferri G, Corradini B, Ferrari F, Santunione AL, Palazzoli F, Alu M. Forensic botany II, DNA barcode for land plants: Which markers after the international agreement? Forensic Science International: Genetics. 2015;**15**:131-136. DOI: 10.1016/j.fsigen.2014.10.005

[30] Meyer R, Chardonnens F, Hübner P, Lüthy J. Polymerase chain reaction (PCR) in the quality and safety assurance of food: Detection of soya in

processed meat products. Zeitschrift für Lebensmittel-Untersuchung und Forschung. 1996;**203**:339-344. DOI: 10.1007/BF01231072

[31] Taberlet P, Gielly L, Pautou G, Bouvet J. Universal primers for amplification of three noncoding regions of chloroplast DNA. Plant Molecular Biology. 1991;**17**:1105-1109. DOI: 10.1007/BF00037152

[32] Gierson E, Tucker GA, Keen J, Ray J, Bird CR, Schuch W. Sequencing and identification of a cDNA clone for tomato polygalacturonase. Nucleic Acid Research. 1986;**14**:8595-8603. DOI: 10.1093/nar/14.21.8595

[33] Pietsch K, Waiblinger HU, Brodmann P, Wurz A. Screening methods for the identification of "genetically modified" food of plant origin. Deutsche Lebensmittel Rundschau. 1997;**93**:35-38

[34] Hemmer W. Foods derived from genetically modified organisms and detection methods. In: BATS Report by Centre for Biosafety and Sustainability. Basel, Switzerland; 1997. pp. 40-44

[35] Wolf C, Scherzinger M, Wurz A, Pauli U, Hübner P, Lüthy J. Detection of cauliflower mosaic virus by the polymerase chain reaction: Testing of food components for false-positive 35S-promoter screening results. European Food Research and Technology. 2000;**210**:367-372. DOI: 10.1007/s002170050565

[36] Deisingh AK, Badrie N. Detection approaches for genetically modified organisms in foods. Food Research International. 2005;**38**:639-649. DOI: 10.1016/j.foodres.2005.01.003

[37] Holst-Jensen A. Testing for genetically modified organisms (GMOs): Past, present and future perspectives. Biotechnology Advances. 2009;**27**:1071-1082. DOI: 10.1016/j.biotechadv.2009.05.025

[38] Southern EM. Detection of specific sequences among DNA fragments separated by gel electrophoresis. Journal of Molecular Biology. 1975;**98**:503-517. DOI: 10.1016/S0022-2836(75)80083-0

[39] Leimanis S, Hernández M, Fernández S, Boyer F, Burns M, Bruderer S, et al. A microarray-based detection system for genetically modified (GM) food ingredients. Plant Molecular Biology. 2006;**61**:123-139. DOI: 10.1007/s11103-005-6173-4

[40] Kim JH, Kim SY, Lee H, Kim YR, Kim HY. An event-specific DNA microarray to identify genetically modified organisms in processed foods. Journal of Agriculture and Food Chemistry. 2010;**58**:6018-6026. DOI: 10.1021/jf100351x

[41] Elenis DS, Kalogianni DP, Glynou K, Ioannou PC, Christopoulos TK. Advances in molecular techniques for the detection and quantification of genetically modified organisms. Analytical and Bioanalytical Chemistry. 2008;**392**:347-354. DOI: 10.1007/s00216-008-1868-4

[42] Querci M, Bulcke MV, Jana Ž, Guy VE, Hermann B. New approaches in GMO detection. Analytical and Bioanalytical Chemistry. 2010;**396**:1991-2002. DOI: 10.1007/s00216-009-3237-3

[43] Von Gotz F. See what you eat--Broad GMO screening with microarrays. Analytical and Bioanalytical Chemistry. 2010;**396**:1961-1970. DOI: 10.1007/s00216-009-3204-z

[44] Heid CA, Stevens J, Livak KJ, Williams PM. Real time quantitative PCR. Genome Research. 1996;**6**:986-994. DOI: 10.1101/gr.6.10.986

[45] Higuchi R, Fockler C, Dollinger G, Watson R. Kinetic PCR analysis:

Real time monitoring of DNA amplification reactions. Biotechnology. 1993;**11**:1026-1030. DOI: 10.1038/nbt0993-1026

[46] Ferreira JL, Geraldo MAC, Aluízio B, Wellington SG, Tesfahun AS. Biosafety and detection of genetically modified organisms. In: Çiftçi YO, editor. Transgenic Plants—Advances and Limitations. Intecopen; 2012. pp. 427-448. DOI: 10.13140/RG.2.1.3470.2245

[47] Brett GM, Chambers SJ, Huang L, Morgan MRA. Design and development of immunoassays for detection of proteins. Food Control. 1999;**10**:401-406. DOI: 10.1016/S0956-7135(99)00082-1

[48] Conceição FR, Moreira AN, Binsfeld PC. Detecção de organismos geneticamente modificados em alimentos e ingredientes alimentares. Ciência Rural. 2004;**36**:315-324. DOI: 10.1590/S0103-84782006000100053

[49] Urbanek-Karlowska B, Fonberg-Broczek M, Sawilska-Rautenstrauch D, Badowski P, Jedra M. Usefulness of an immunoassay test trait for detection of genetically modified roundup ready soybean in food products. Rocz Panstwowy Zaklad Higieny. 2001;**52**:313-320

[50] Lipton CR, Dautlick JX, Grothaus GD, Hunst PL, Magin KM, Mihaliak CA, et al. Guidelines for the validation and use of immunoassays for determining of introduced proteins in biotechnology enhanced crops and derived food ingredients. Food and Agriculture Immunology. 2000;**12**:153-164. DOI: 10.1080/095401000404094

[51] Kuiper HA. Summary report of the ILSI Europe workshop on detection methods for novel foods derived from genetically modified organisms. Food Control. 1999;**10**:339-349. DOI: 10.1016/S0956-7135(99)00072-9

[52] Ahmed FE. Detection of genetically modified organisms in foods. Trends in Biotechnology. 2002;**20**:215-223. DOI: 10.1016/S0167-7799(01)01920-5

[53] Serageldin I. Biotechnology and food security in the 21st century. Science. 1999;**285**:387-389. DOI: 10.1126/science.285.5426.387

[54] Areal FJ, Riesgo L, Rodriguez-Cerezo E. Economic and agronomic impact of commercialized GM crops: A meta analysis. The Journal of Agricultural Science. 2013;**151**:7-33. DOI: 10.1017/S0021859612000111

[55] Finger R, El Benni N, Kaphengst T, Evans C, Herbert S, Lehmann B, et al. A meta analysis on farm-level costs and benefits of GM crops. Sustainability. 2011;**3**:743-762. DOI: 10.3929/ethz-b-000042242

[56] Brookes G, Barfoot P. Global income and production impacts of using GM crop technology. 1996-2014. GM Crops and Food. 2016;**7**:38-77. DOI: 10.1080/21645698.2016.1176817

[57] Ives AR, Cate P, Andrew H, Sharon D, David AA, Ralph H, et al. Spatio-temporal variation in landscape composition may speed resistance evolution of pests to Bt crops. PLoS One. 2017;**12**:e0169167. DOI: 10.1371/journal.pone.01691675

[58] Finamore A, Marianna R, Serena B, Giovanni M, Roberto A, Aida T, et al. Intestinal and peripheral immune response to Mon810 maize ingestion in weaning and old mice. Journal of Agricultural and Food Chemistry. 2008;**56**:11533-11539. DOI: 10.1021/jf802059w

[59] Economic Survey of Pakistan 2017-18. Chapter-2 Agriculture, Economic Adviser's Wing, Finance Division, Government of Pakistan. pp. 13-32

[60] ISAAA. Global Status of Commercialized Biotech/GM Crops: 2016. ISAAA Brief No. 52. Ithaca, New York: ISAAA; 2016

[61] Gabol WA, Ahmed A, Bux H, Ahmed K, Mahar A, Laghari S. Genetically modified organisms (GMOs) in Pakistan. African Journal of Biotechnology. 2012;**11**:2807-2813. DOI: 10.5897/AJBX11.001

[62] Khan MS, Joyia FA. Biotechnology and GM crops. In: Khan IA, Khan MS, editors. Developing Sustainable Agriculture in Pakistan. Taylor and Francis, USA: CRC PressTaylor and Francis; 2018. pp. 355-368